A BETTER BIRTH

10 WAYS TO REDUCE YOUR CHANCE OF HAVING A CESAREAN BIRTH

BY

JENNIFER MORE

A Dolphin Method Publication

PUBLISHER'S NOTE

This publication is designed to provide accurate and authoritative information in regard to the subject matter covered. It is sold with the understanding that the publisher is not engaged in providing medical, psychological, physical, emotional, or professional services. If expert or medical assistance is needed, the services of a competent professional should be sought.

Dolphin Method Publishing
Santa Rosa, California
info@dolphinmethod.com
www.dolphinmethod.com

Cover Design: Marta Dec
Interior Design: Erin Teh, Jake More
Publisher: Dolphin Method Publications
Editor: Michael Shapiro, Lucy Loscocco
Creative Consultant: Jake More
ISBN: 978-1-7328967-5-8
Library of Congress Control Number: 2018912433
VXFB - Pregnancy, Birth, and Baby Care
First Edition

THIS BOOK IS DEDICATED TO MY DAUGHTER SYDNEY WHOSE BIRTH CHANGED MY LIFE AND SET ME ON THE PATH I AM ON TODAY.

THANK YOU

I would like to thank my husband Jake and amazing daughters Sydney and Ella who are the lights of my life. I want to thank them for their support and belief in me all these years and for putting up with a career that takes me away for days or weeks at a time. Also a huge thank you to my parents Joan and Richard for being role models for me throughout my life as authors and teachers themselves they have always inspired me and encouraged me to follow my dreams, even when they weren't sure where they would lead! And to my sister Liz Rossi who is there for me 24/7 believing in me even when I didn't believe in myself. And my wonderful in laws Gae and Michael who have been and continue to be incredibly supportive.

I would also like to extend a thank you to all of the birth professionals who work with pregnant and postpartum women that I have been so fortunate to know and who have inspired me through the years. Specifically, Melissa French who took the time to give me valuable input on this book. And lastly thank you to all the women and families who have given me the privilege of attending their births and helping them through the journey of childbirth.

Jennifer Mare

CONTENTS

Introduction 8

Chapter 1   **Choose your Birth Location and Birth Team Wisely** 16

Birth facility and care provider options
Choosing a birth facility and a care provider
Effects on birth outcomes using a doula

Chapter 2   **Childbirth Education** 28

Hospital childbirth education classes
Private and small group childbirth education classes
Online childbirth education classes

Chapter 3   **Optimal Fetal Positions During Pregnancy** 34

Fetal positions
What is the optimal fetal position?
Breech and transverse babies
Positions and techniques for turning breech babies
Positions to avoid

Chapter 4   **Yoga** 48

The Dolphin Method 15-minute practice

Chapter 5   **Avoid Induction** 62

Most common reasons for induction
What is induction and how is it done?
Risks of medical inductions
Use your B.R.A.I.N.
Natural methods of induction

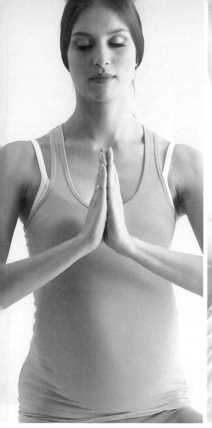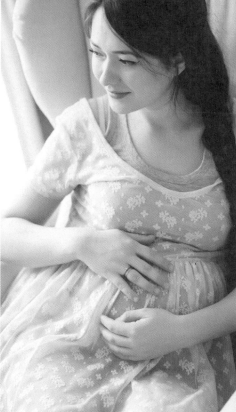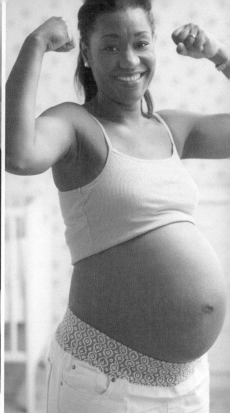

Chapter 6   **Create Your Environment** 74

Optimizing your external environment
Optimizing your internal environment

Chapter 7   **Labor at Home Longer** 82

Chapter 8   **Avoid Early Epidural and Other Interventions** 92

What is an epidural?
When is the best time to get an epidural?
Relaxation techniques – physical
Relaxation techniques – emotional

Chapter 9   **Pelvic Opening: Movements Specific to Labor** 102

Chapter 10   **Sensation Control: Believe in your body** 112

How do we redefine sensation?

Final Thoughts 124

Glossary of Terms 125

Notes 128

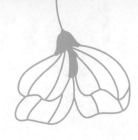

INTRODUCTION

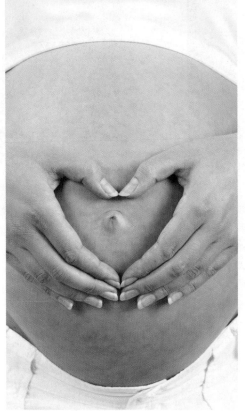

The amazing process of pregnancy and childbirth reveals the profound potential that lies within each of us. It is beautiful in so many ways and has the potential to be an empowering, joyful and transformative journey. My life's work is helping women prepare for and embrace their pregnant bodies to help them have positive, ecstatic birth experiences that prove to them that they can do anything, that they are powerful, strong and capable.

I'd like to thank you for reading this book and choosing to become an active participant in your pregnancy and childbirth experience. These days, you are presented with myriad choices and opinions as you begin to explore the realities of pregnancy and childbirth. The choices begin as soon as you discover that you are pregnant and can have lifelong consequences for you and for your child. The options for most women are numerous and confusing, and it is very easy to become overwhelmed and want to take the path of least resistance. The problem with that path is that it can lead to outcomes that you may not be happy with, and that's where this book comes in. Although the title of this book is *10 Ways To Reduce Your Chance of Having a Cesarean Birth*, its main purpose is to help you with some of these decisions so that you are prepared to have a birth experience that is positive, regardless of the ultimate method of delivering your baby.

Before we dive into the ten ways to reduce your chance of having a cesarean, I would like to acknowledge with extreme gratitude the contribution that science and medicine have made to the field of childbirth with regard to delivering babies via cesarean. I would also like to acknowledge that in certain circumstances cesareans are very appropriate and save lives. Although this book is designed to help you have the best chance of avoiding a cesarean, it is also important that we acknowledge that sometimes cesareans are medically necessary for the health of the mom and the baby.

My hope is that if you end up needing a cesarean, you will know that you've done everything you can to give yourself the best opportunity for a vaginal delivery and can ultimately embrace the experience of cesarean birth with gratitude rather than disappointment or a sense of failure. With that said, the consensus of the World Health Organization and many others is that cesareans have higher risks to both mom and baby and are performed far more often than medically necessary. The World Health Organization states: "There is no justification for any region to have CS rates higher than 10-15 percent".[1]

I'd like to share a story that suggests how the information in this book can help even if you end up having a cesarean. I was attending my very first birth as a doula, many years ago. My client went into labor at 35 weeks. Based on the baby's gestational age, she was allowed to labor for quite a long time, because they wanted the baby to be as mature as possible when he was born. I was with her for 64 hours straight. We tried every method that I knew at the time. We tried different positions. We did hypnosis and relaxation techniques. We even had an acupuncturist come into the labor and delivery room to try to help turn the baby. After all of this work and effort, the midwife and doctor finally came in and said that the baby was not doing well and that the mother needed to have a cesarean. This being my first birth as a doula, I was devastated. I felt like I had failed. I was so far beyond tired that I was thinking to myself, "I cannot do this work. I put in all of this time, yet it meant nothing because she's still having a cesarean." They wheeled her out of the room to prepare her for the surgery, and I was left in her room alone until I heard her call my name from the hall. I ran out to see what she needed. I remember her lying there and turning her head to look at me. She said, "Jennifer, I just want you to know, I had a really great birth experience." I went back into her room and cried because I was exhausted. I cried because she was having a cesarean, but I mostly cried because I had made a difference. This experience that could have been traumatic and disillusioning for her was ultimately positive, because she knew she had done everything she could possibly have done to avoid having a cesarean. There was no doubt in her mind that she needed it. The impact of this birth changed the way I viewed success and failure in birth.

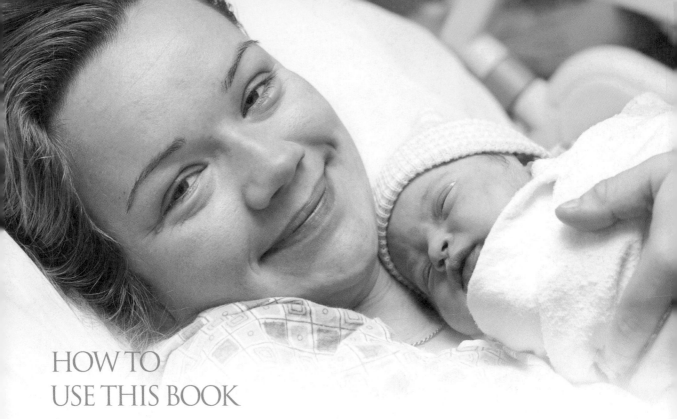

HOW TO
USE THIS BOOK

My goal in writing this book is for you to have an easy-to-read but comprehensive guide to help you have the best birth experience possible.

Because there are so many great childbirth education resources out there, I don't want to spend a lot of time educating you about everything you'll need to know. However, you will encounter many medical terms and procedures with which you may not be familiar, so I have created a supplemental website that you can turn to that offers additional information.

You will see various icons to let you know that you will find supporting information about that word or topic online or in the book.

Visit: www.dolphinmethod.com/resources

 This icon indicates there is supporting information on the website

 This icon indicates there is a definition of the term in the glossary at the end of the book, as well as on the website

 This icon indicates that you should seek approval from your doctor or midwife before attempting a specific physical activity

 This icon indicates that you can perform a specific pose in the bed as well as on the floor

WHY DO WE WANT TO AVOID CESAREANS?

In addition to learning ways to avoid cesareans, I think it is important that women are aware of the risks of this procedure. Cesareans are major abdominal surgery and need to be respected as such. Cultures in many modernized societies have normalized cesareans as just another birth option. In some cultures, women choose this surgery as a form of status or a way to protect their perineum from the harm of vaginal delivery. In this chapter, we will discuss some of the risks of cesarean surgery so that you are empowered to make an informed decision regarding your childbirth.

Many women decide they want a cesarean to avoid the pain of childbirth. However it is important to understand that having a cesarean does not necessarily mean you'll have less pain. Studies show[2] that 80 percent of women who have had cesareans have moderate to severe pain and after two years, a third of those with pain experienced chronic pain at the incision site. Of these women with chronic pain, 7 percent reported severe pain and 8.9 percent had pain that impaired their daily activities. The conclusion of this study was that chronic pain occurs commonly after bikini-cut cesareans. Nerve entrapment was found to be one of the main causes of moderate to severe pain. As well as pain, we also see many women having numbness or loss of feeling in the incision area as well as referred pain in the back, neck, abdomen or pelvic area.

Prominent medical institutions, including the National Institutes of Health, the World Health Organization, The Centers for Disease Control and Prevention, and the American Congress of Obstetrics and Gynecology (ACOG), have researched the risks of cesarean delivery. These risks are not the same due to varying protocols, safety standards and surgical techniques used in different parts of the world. Some general findings are listed below.

ACOG's list of possible maternal cesarean complications[3] includes

- Increased risk of infection
- Increased risk of re-hospitalization within 30 days of surgery
- Blood loss
- Blood clots in the legs, pelvic organs or lungs
- Injury to the bowel or bladder
- Reaction to medications or anesthesia used

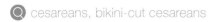 cesareans, bikini-cut cesareans

The National Institutes of Health adds to these findings[4]

- Infants delivered by pre-labor cesarean were nearly 7 times as likely to develop respiratory morbidity. This included deliveries between 37 and 42 weeks gestation. This risk, however, decreased after 39 weeks.
- Fetal laceration occurs in 0.1 – 3.1 percent of cesarean deliveries.
- A 2008 study finds a 20 percent increase in the risk of asthma in children who had been delivered by cesarean section.[5]
- Several theories are being studied and substantiated about the relationship between cesareans and increases in childhood allergies, asthma and autoimmune diseases. The correlation can be found in the gut microbiota of the intestines of babies birthed via cesarean versus vaginal delivery.[6]
- Longer recovery time

The Centers for Disease Control and Prevention finds[7] cesareans are associated with increased risk of:

- Maternal transfusion
- Ruptured uterus
- Unplanned hysterectomy
- Admission to Intensive Care Unit

Other risks of cesareans that are commonly discussed in the birth community are higher risks of ectopic pregnancies, higher percentages of placenta praevia and placental abruption in future pregnancies and long-term pain or numbness in the scar area as well as chronic back, abdominal or pelvic pain.

gut microbiota, Maternal transfusion, hysterectomy, placenta praevia, placental abruption

MATERNAL MORBIDITY FOR VAGINAL AND CESAREAN DELIVERIES, ACCORDING TO PREVIOUS CESAREAN HISTORY: NEW DATA FROM THE BIRTH CERTIFICATES, 2013

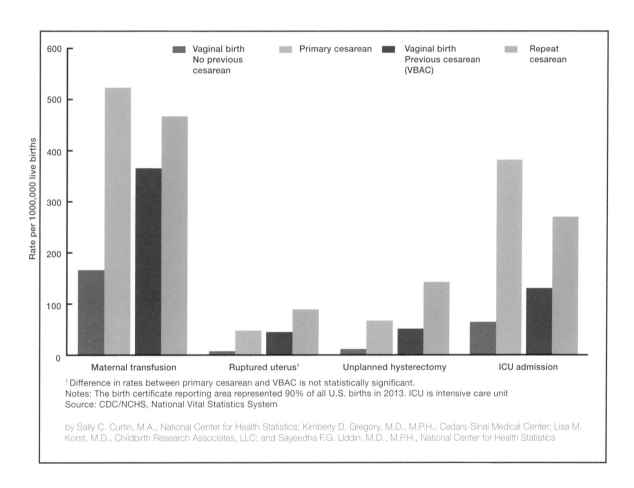

[1] Difference in rates between primary cesarean and VBAC is not statistically significant.
Notes: The birth certificate reporting area represented 90% of all U.S. births in 2013. ICU is intensive care unit
Source: CDC/NCHS, National Vital Statistics System

by Sally C. Curtin, M.A., National Center for Health Statistics; Kimberly D. Gregory, M.D., M.P.H., Cedars-Sinai Medical Center; Lisa M. Korst, M.D., Childbirth Research Associates, LLC; and Sayeedha F.G. Uddin, M.D., M.P.H., National Center for Health Statistics

VAGINAL BIRTH AFTER CESAREAN (VBAC) AND TRIAL OF LABOR AFTER CESAREAN (TOLAC)

Let's talk for a minute about vaginal births after cesarean. Women who have had a previous cesarean and are thinking about having a vaginal birth (VBAC), or women who wish to have a trial of labor after cesarean (TOLAC), can also benefit from the information in this book. By the way, the woman mentioned in the story above went on to have a vaginal delivery a few years later. If this is the case for you, you need to be aware of a few things.

The American Congress of Obstetrics and Gynecology (ACOG) now recommends VBAC or TOLAC for most low-risk women with a few exceptions.[8] Those exceptions are:

- If you have had a high vertical incision in a previous cesarean
- If you have had a prior uterine rupture
- If you have a medical condition that makes vaginal delivery risky
- If you are at a hospital that is not prepared to deal with emergencies that may arise

American College Of Gynecology further encourages Vaginal Birth After Cesarean because it is associated with some maternal benefits compared to a planned cesarean delivery.

These include:

- No abdominal surgery
- Shorter recovery period
- Lower risk of infection
- Less blood loss

They go on to mention that women who may want to have more children may benefit from VBAC because it will help them avoid problems associated with multiple cesarean deliveries. The problems they acknowledge are a higher risk of hysterectomy, bowel or bladder injury and certain problems with the placenta. If you are considering a VBAC, I recommend researching your birth facility and options that exist in your area as well as having a conversation with your doctor about your particular situation. I encourage you to get a second opinion if you don't feel comfortable with the outcome of this conversation.

With this information in mind, let's begin exploring ways that you can empower yourself to have the best birth experience possible and reduce your chance of having a cesarean birth.

Chapter 1

CHOOSE YOUR
BIRTH LOCATION
AND
BIRTH TEAM
WISELY

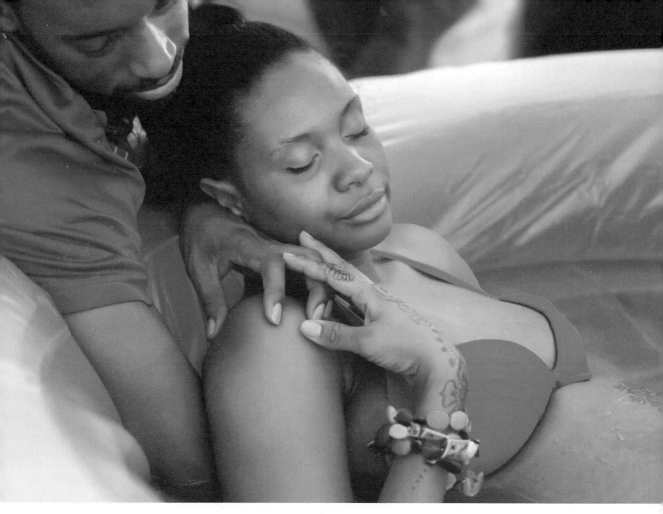

WHERE YOU CHOOSE TO HAVE YOUR BABY AND WHOM YOU CHOOSE AS YOUR CARE PROVIDER CAN MAKE A HUGE DIFFERENCE IN THE KIND OF BIRTH EXPERIENCE AND BIRTH OUTCOME YOU HAVE.

This chapter will explore some things to look for in a birth location as well as in a doctor or midwife. Some of you may have limited options depending on where you live or the type of insurance you have, while others have a multitude of choices. So let's explore the things you can do regardless of any possible limitations.

 midwife

BIRTH FACILITY AND CARE PROVIDER OPTIONS

Where do you envision welcoming your baby into the world? Depending on where you live, you might have several options about where to deliver your baby, so let's look at the most popular options:

HOSPITALS

In many modern cities around the world, hospitals are the most common places to deliver babies. Some are more progressive than others when it comes to birth. They might include birth centers adjacent to or inside of hospitals, many of which are attended mainly by midwives with doctors on call in case they are needed. Some hospitals might be better suited to high-risk pregnancies, while others might offer labor suites with bathtubs in them.

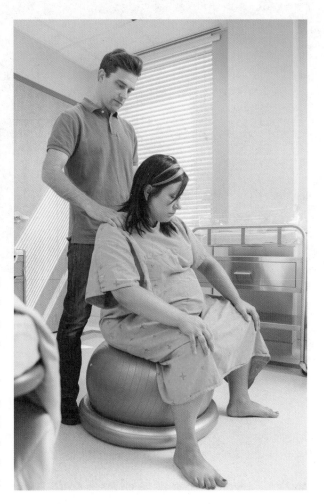

BIRTH CENTERS

Freestanding birth centers are commonly attended by midwives and sometimes include support by doulas. They typically have an obstetrician on call and a hospital nearby in case transfer to the hospital is medically necessary. Most of the time, women giving birth at a birth center are looking for a more natural experience with few interventions and the security that there is a hospital nearby and a staff at the birth center who is knowledgeable and supportive. Countries that use birth centers and home birth options tend to have the lowest cesarean rates.

doula   birth centers

HOME BIRTH

In some places, women may have the option to deliver their babies at home with the assistance of a midwife. This can be a good option for low-risk women who are looking for a more natural experience than they would get at a hospital, with few to no interventions, and the ability to give birth the way they want, where they are most comfortable.

Because options vary widely from place to place, it is best that you do some research on options in your area and see what is available to you. Explore all your options, even if they don't seem feasible or desirable. In researching them, you might change your mind about what you want.

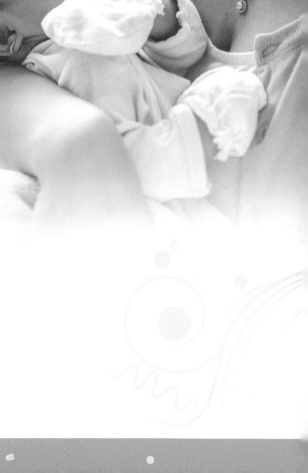

CHOOSING A BIRTH FACILITY AND A CARE PROVIDER

LOCATION

How far do you live from the facility?

Labor is unpredictable. The average first-time labor is about 24 hours, giving you lots of time to get to a faraway hospital or birth location, but that is the average time, not the expected time. Your labor could be only 45 minutes long, or it could take several days. Because we have no way to know the length of your labor ahead of time, it is best to be able to get to your birth facility quickly. This is not only because of the chance of not making it in time for your baby to be born, but also because traveling while in labor is not the most enjoyable experience. If you find that the ideal place for you to give birth is a bit far away, see if there is somewhere you could stay when you first feel labor starting that is closer to the facility, and make that trip early in labor. Also make sure that if you choose a location that is far away from you that you have multiple options to help you get there when you need to go.

AMENITIES AND INTERVENTIONS

What are the standard practices at the hospital or birth center, and what amenities are offered and widely used? Not all hospitals and birth facilities are created equal. You will want to tour the facility if possible.

Here are some things to inquire about when researching hospitals and other birth facilities:

- How long are you able to stay after the delivery for a vaginal birth or a cesarean delivery?
- What is the facility's cesarean rate? The rates of cesareans differ greatly from birth centers to hospitals and from hospital to hospital (even within a few miles of each other). If you can find out the cesarean rates of the birth facilities in your area, I recommend doing so.
- How many rooms are there and how many women (on average) give birth there each day?
- How many people can be in the room with you, and are there times when your partner must leave the room?
- Do they allow you to bring a doula or labor coach?
- Can you freely eat and drink while in labor?

- Do they insist that every woman has an IV upon entering the facility?
- What are their rates of women using pain medication and what kinds are offered?
- Are there bathtubs or showers in each room? If so, what is the policy around using them?
- What is the policy about maternal and fetal monitoring; how often is it done?
- Can you freely move around in the room, if un-medicated, and utilize different positions during labor, pushing, and delivery?
- If the facility is not a hospital, what is their rate of women needing a transfer to the hospital?
- Are the labor rooms private or shared?
- Are the delivery rooms private or shared?
- What are the policies after the baby is born?
- Can the baby be placed directly on mom's skin after delivery?
- Can the cutting of the umbilical cord be delayed?
- Can you take the placenta home?
- What are the newborn tests and procedures?
- Can the baby skip the first bath if desired by mom?
- Is there breastfeeding support immediately postpartum and before the mom is discharged?
- Is there a NICU (neonatal intensive care unit)? If not, where will the baby be transferred if there is a health concern?
- Does the baby stay in the room with mom after delivery? Is there a time when babies are taken to the nursery?
- What are the policies for visitors?

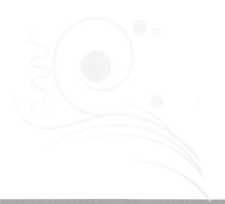

THE DOCTOR, MIDWIFE OR OTHER CARE PROVIDER

The care provider you choose is just as, if not more, important than the birth facility. Your care provider plays an important role in your ability to feel safe and cared for during your pregnancy and labor. They also need to be able to assist you if interventions are needed as you are delivering your baby. If you have a choice of care providers, I highly recommend that you interview several, and see which ones you connect with the best. If you are contemplating a home birth, look for midwives who serve the area where you live. If you have already chosen a birth facility, look at the doctors or midwives who are associated with that facility first. Don't be afraid to have a conversation with your prospective doctor or midwife! They are just people, and building rapport with them is a good way to be given more leeway when it comes time to deliver your baby. During your visits, treat them like you would a formal friend. Ask them how their day has been; get them talking with you, so they remember who you are and look forward to your visits. Also when you ask them questions, use a pleasant tone of voice. Don't demand anything, but inquire from a strong place of knowledge. If they say something you don't like or aren't comfortable with, ask them to explain their thinking about it. If you still don't agree, tell them in a nice way that you would like to explore other possibilities, and open a line of communication with them.

Remember that you are the consumer, and they are working for you! Doctors and midwives are in a business. If there is a demand for things to be a certain way with birth and there are other doctors or midwives willing to fill that demand, they will eventually have to fill it or patients will stop coming to them. So, even if you live in a place where the birth environment is very conservative or medicalized, asking for what you want is an important way to begin to see change.

Here are some of the questions you might want to ask a prospective doctor or midwife:

- How often will I see you for appointments, and where will they be?
- Do you insist that every laboring woman has an IV?
- How do you feel about eating and drinking while in labor, if I am hungry?
- When labor begins, or I think it is, when should I call you?
- How long are you comfortable with me staying at home laboring:
  - With water intact?
  - With water broken?

- For what reasons do you perform the following, and what are your statistics for each:
  - An episiotomy?
  - A cesarean section?
  - Vacuum or forceps delivery?
- What percentage of your patients are medicated during the birth?
- Are you comfortable with me laboring out of bed?
- In what positions are you comfortable having me push and deliver the baby?
- Assuming everything is good with the baby and myself, how long can I go past my due date before you would want to induce labor?
- How do you feel about natural induction techniques such as acupuncture?
- If you are not on call, who is your primary backup?
- How many people will you allow in the labor room?
- Can my support person stay with me if/when I have an epidural or cesarean (how many in the operating room for a cesarean)?

TESTIMONIALS

The best way to find a good healthcare provider or birth facility is to talk to people who have had positive experiences or are part of the larger birth community. I recommend talking to local doulas, prenatal yoga teachers, childbirth educators, or midwives. They will likely know the birth-friendly doctors and hospitals in your area. If nothing else, you can always ask friends who have had positive experiences where and with whom they delivered.

HIRE A DOULA

To round out your birth team, I highly recommend hiring a doula. There are several different kinds of doulas. What is a doula? Birth doulas work with women before, during and after the birth of their babies to help ensure a safe and satisfying birth experience. They typically meet with the pregnant woman a couple of times to build rapport, so the woman feels safe with them.

Doulas provide emotional support and physical comfort and facilitate communication with the medical staff to make sure laboring women have the information necessary to make educated decisions during childbirth. They provide reassurance and perspective to the laboring woman and her partner, making suggestions for labor progress and supporting her with comfort techniques that may include relaxation, massage, positioning, and touch. Doulas are usually independent contractors working for the laboring woman, not the caregiver or hospital. There are some hospitals and birth centers that now utilize doulas and have them available for those who want them.

Having a doula can take some of the fear out of the birth experience, helping you feel more comfortable, safe, and nurtured. The doula may be the only other person at the labor who is there exclusively for the emotional well being of the mom. Most of the time, doulas offer continuous care from the beginning of labor through the birth of the baby and sometimes beyond.

This may mean going to the mother's house and following her to the hospital or birth center when labor begins. Other people who are present on and off during labor and delivery, such as the nurse, doctor or midwife, are concerned for the mother but also have other responsibilities and priorities that may compete with the birthing woman's emotional needs. They have to make sure hospital policies are maintained. They have shift changes and need to continuously focus on the well being of the baby. The only priority the doula has is the mother. She stays through shift changes, helps the woman through each contraction and supports the family so that the partner can be as involved as they would like to be without the concern of having to know what to do next.

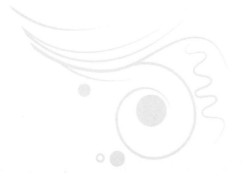

Here are some important questions to ask a perspective doula:

- Why did you become a doula and what is your philosophy regarding supporting women and families through the birth experience?
- How do you work as a doula?
  - When should I call you?
  - When do you show up after labor begins?
  - Do you meet with me/us prior to the birth? How many times and for how long?
  - Should my partner be present?
  - Do you do a visit after the birth? If so, how soon?
- What kind of training or certification do you have?
  - Tell me about your experience.
  - Do you work in hospitals? Which ones?
  - Do you attend home births or birth center births?
  - Are there certain doctors or midwives you've worked with regularly or hospitals and birth locations you frequent?
- What is your fee?
  - Do you require a deposit?
  - What is your fee schedule?
  - What is your refund policy?
- What is your availability?
  - How do you schedule clients?
  - Do you have a backup doula(s)?
  - Under which circumstances do you use them?
  - Can I/we meet them?
- Will you discuss a birth plan or early labor plan with me and help me come up with an appropriate one?
- Do you offer any additional services like placental encapsulation, massage, hypnosis, etc.?
- Do you have any references I can contact?

The most important thing to consider before you hire a doula is whether or not you feel safe and connected with her. A doula will be with you during one of the most intimate and vulnerable times of your life, so chemistry matters more than years of experience! Interview several doulas if possible and choose the one who best fits your personality.

I recommend the book *Mothering the Mother: How a Doula Can Help You Have a Shorter, Easier, and Healthier Birth* by Marshall H. Klaus, M.D.; John H. Kennell, M.D.; and Phyllis H. Klaus, M. Ed., C.S.W. In this book they published the following statistics about doulas and the effects on birth outcomes:

EFFECTS ON BIRTH OUTCOMES USING A DOULA

Although birth outcomes vary for many reasons, studies have shown that when using a doula, women have had:

- Labors are 25 percent shorter
- Cesarean rates are reduced by 50 percent
- There is 40 percent less need for oxytocin to speed up labor
- Need for forceps is reduced by 40 percent
- Women request 30 percent less pain medication and 60 percent fewer epidurals

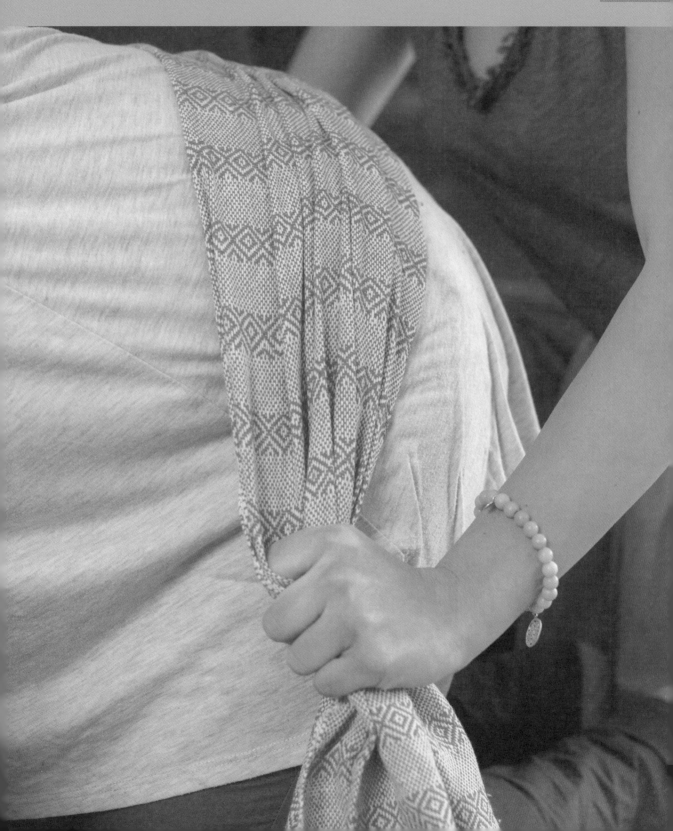

CHILDBIRTH
EDUCATION

PARTICIPATING IN A HIGHLY REGARDED CHILDBIRTH EDUCATION CLASS CAN PLAY AN IMPORTANT ROLE IN HELPING YOU HAVE A POSITIVE BIRTH EXPERIENCE AND REDUCE THE LIKELIHOOD OF HAVING A CESAREAN.[9]

Childbirth classes can help you understand the process the body goes through during labor and childbirth and the options you have to make the experience one that is right for you. They describe the stages, anatomy and physiology of labor and childbirth and teach you what to expect from your body and the environment during each stage of labor (hospital protocols/staff responses). Childbirth classes also describe the risks and benefits of different widely used medical interventions. Specialized childbirth education classes also give a pregnant woman and her partner tools and techniques to help with the fear and discomfort of childbirth.

Childbirth education has grown over the years from exclusively teaching about labor and delivery to sometimes including teaching about caring for your newborn, breastfeeding, and other relevant pre- and postnatal topics. Depending on where you live, there may be several options available. Here are some tips to find the best available childbirth education class.

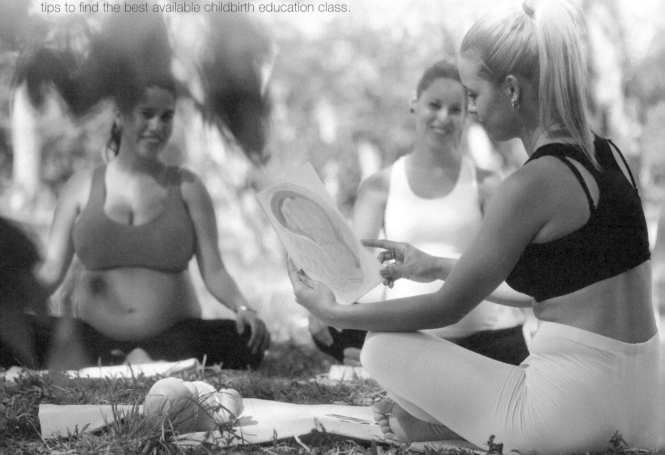

HOSPITAL
CHILDBIRTH EDUCATION CLASSES

Childbirth education classes offered by hospitals are becoming more popular all over the world. They are usually the most convenient and affordable live classes for women or couples. It is hard to lump them all into one category since they are so different, depending on the individual hospital and teacher. Hospital classes typically run anywhere from a one-day course of approximately 6 to 7 hours to a six-week course running approximately 20 to 30 hours, with many variations in between. Longer classes tend to include more than just the anatomy and physiology of birth; they teach techniques and provide tools to help with pain management. Some offer newborn and initial breastfeeding guidance. These classes tend to appeal to women seeking a natural experience with few interventions.

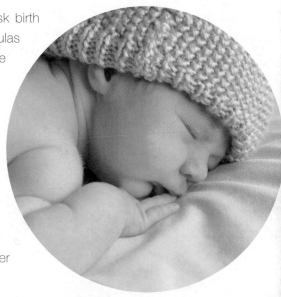

It is a good idea to research hospitals in your area and ask birth professionals (such as local prenatal yoga teachers, doulas or midwives) their impressions of hospital classes you are considering before signing up. Be careful of classes that feel like they have an agenda, for example if you feel more afraid during or after the class or if the class seems to be focusing on topics in a biased way, not giving risks and benefits or explaining all options. Because classes vary so much, I recommend reading a good childbirth book before taking the class, so you come in with questions and know you are getting the information you need. Because childbirth classes are usually taught based on the procedures and policies of the hospital where they are held, you will get to know whether your choice of hospital really suits your desires.

PRIVATE AND SMALL GROUP CHILDBIRTH EDUCATION CLASSES

There are so many different kinds of childbirth education classes out there that it is impossible to list all of your choices here. However, I will bring up a few of the most popular options, so that you have a starting point to look for what's available in your area. The first place I recommend looking for private childbirth education classes is through local birth resource centers or online databases. Also check if there are local mother's clubs or places pregnant women or new moms tend to gather. If those aren't available or useful, reach out to local doulas, midwives, or prenatal yoga teachers. They are likely to be not only your best resource but many of them teach the classes themselves. These classes are typically longer than the hospital classes, though not always, and many of them focus on emotional as well as physical ways of creating positive birth experiences. Some of these classes have a very strong propensity towards natural childbirth. However, a good class will be balanced, providing useful information on ways to have a positive birth experience regardless of the use of medications and intervention. *These classes should empower you to feel like there is no way to fail at giving birth, that your body was made to do this, and give you tools to reduce fear and anxiety.*

HERE ARE SOME THINGS TO LOOK FOR IN A GOOD PRIVATE OR SMALL-GROUP CHILDBIRTH EDUCATION CLASS:

1. Is the teacher inclusive of everyone regardless of what kind of birth the woman is planning to have?

2. Can you find positive testimonials from other women who have taken the class?

3. How many students typically attend the classes?

4. What is the fee and schedule of the class, and how many total hours does it include?

5. What is the educational background of the teacher?

6. Where are classes held, and who is invited to participate *(partner or husband as well as pregnant woman)*?

7. What are the specific topics that will be covered?

8. Is the teacher familiar with the hospital or birth facility where you are planning to deliver your baby?

One of the most recognizable names in childbirth education is Lamaze International; they have trainers in many countries. This might be a good place to look if you are having trouble finding local resources.[10]

ONLINE CHILDBIRTH EDUCATION CLASSES

With so much information available online these days, you have to carefully select and scrutinize the material you find. With proper research, online courses are a good option for those women who find no physical location to take a childbirth class in their area, or who live in remote areas.

The same criteria apply when evaluating online with a few additions.

ONLINE CLASSES

1. Make sure that you can access the class via your computer before paying any money.

2. Check for references and testimonials, aside from what they provide you on their own website.

3. Make sure there is a way for you to ask questions and get answers.

4. Compare the class curriculum of several different courses.

5. Don't look for the quickest and easiest class. Childbirth and labor are dense subjects; if you speed through them, you might be left with unanswered questions. Also classes that are completed in one day or over a weekend don't give you time to digest the information and formulate questions. I recommend an online class that is spread out over several weeks.

 See website for additional information about specific books & childbirth education classes that I recommend.

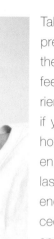

Taking a well researched and comprehensive childbirth class is one of the best things that you can do to feel empowered in your birth experience. This is even more important if you are delivering your baby at a hospital. For most pregnant women, the typical doctor's office visits last only about 5 to 15 minutes, not enough time to learn all of the procedures and policies that you will encounter at the hospital.

Many women I encounter say, "Well I'm just going to have an epidural (pain medication), so I don't really need to know how to cope with childbirth." The truth is, most hospitals won't even admit you until you are in active labor, which could be hours or even days after labor begins! Also, it is important to know that if you get an epidural too early in your labor, your chance of having a cesarean goes up by up to 50 percent. (We will discuss this in detail in a later chapter.) Childbirth education classes can give you the knowledge and tools you need to feel safe during your labor. Those women who feel safe have a lower risk of labor slowing down or stopping, require fewer interventions to keep labor progressing and report having more comfort and less pain throughout the labor process. Surprisingly low numbers of women around the world take childbirth classes, even though the studies directly link these courses to a reduction in cesarean rates.

Chapter 3

Optimal
Fetal
Positions
During
Pregnancy

HOW DOES MOVING YOUR BODY DURING PREGNANCY AFFECT THE POSITION OF YOUR BABY AND IS THAT IMPORTANT?

What is optimal fetal positioning, and why is so important?
Let's explore what it is, then talk a little about what we can do to assist in
achieving and maintaining optimal fetal positioning.

Prior to about 34 weeks of pregnancy, babies have quite a bit
of space to move around. They can change positions often,
though many settle into comfortable positions earlier
and tend to hang out often in the same positions.
After 36 weeks of pregnancy, babies have less room to move around,
so it's beneficial for them to be in an optimal position by then so they have
the easiest path through the pelvis.

Achieving optimal fetal positioning late in pregnancy can be greatly
influenced by what a woman does all the way through pregnancy.

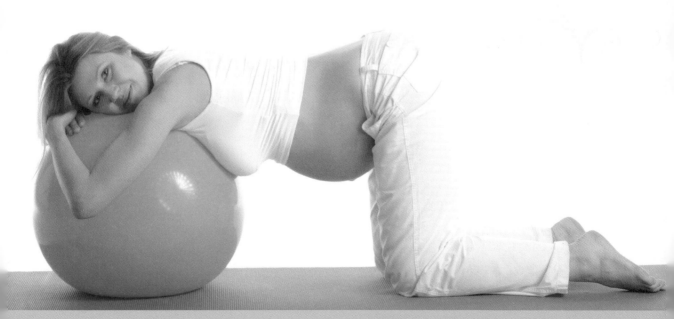

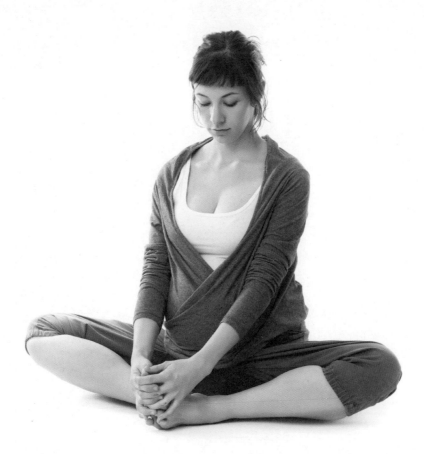

Many women don't understand that in their daily lives, repetitive movements and habitual body positioning can play a major role in what position the baby ends up in when labor begins. The reason for this is that the uterus, where the baby is living and growing, is surrounded on all sides by musculature and bony structures that are influencing its position. The muscles of the pelvic floor, the ligaments that stabilize the uterus and the many muscles and bones that surround it can affect the position in which the baby situates during pregnancy and ultimately affect the ease of the baby's descent through the pelvis during childbirth.

It's all about balance. When all of the ligaments, bones and muscles that surround the uterus are in balance, babies will have a better opportunity to achieve optimal positioning. Optimal positioning is not only helpful for a faster and easier birth but also influences the comfort of the pregnant woman. When the body is in balance, there is less back pain (the most common physical complaint of pregnant women), less hip and pelvic pain and less overall discomfort. Ultimately, ideal fetal positioning is one of the most important aspects of reducing your chance for having a cesarean.

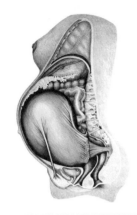

1

Here is a cross section of a pregnant woman's body showing the musculature of the uterus. Notice the connections that attach the uterus to the pelvis. When these structures get out of balance, fetal positioning can be affected.

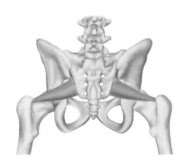

2

The muscle shown here is the piriformas, a key player in pelvic stability and one of the main culprits in back pain for pregnant women.

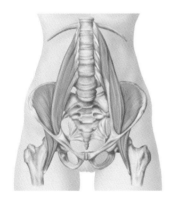

3

This group of muscles is called the iliopsoas, and it sits directly behind the uterus. Too much sitting and imbalance can cause tightness in these muscles and affect the positioning of the uterus and ultimately the fetus.

There are two ways to get in balance and have a positive impact on your baby's position. First is getting your body into positions that encourage balance on a regular basis. Just doing positions once or twice is not going to accomplish much. If you want your body to get into balance, you need to do positions every day that will encourage balance in the body. Second, know which positions in your daily life encourage malposition and avoid them, replacing them with more favorable options.

WHAT IS THE OPTIMAL FETAL POSITION?

Optimal Foetal Positioning (OFP), coined by Jean Sutton and Pauline Scott in *Understanding and Teaching Optimal Foetal Positioning*, is when the baby is in one of the following head down positions: Occipital Anterior, Left Occipital Anterior, or Left Occipital Transverse, often referred to as OA, LOA or LOT (see the chart below.) When the baby moves down through the top opening of the pelvis, LOA is commonly the most preferable and when the baby moves down through the middle and lower parts of the pelvis, OA usually works best. In an LOA or LOT presentation, the baby is head down with the back of the head (the occipital bone) pointing to the left side of the mother or the mother's left front. In the OA presentation the baby is head down, and the back of the head is pointing to the mother's front.

Occipital Anterior position is optimal for a number of reasons. The baby's head molds as it moves through the birth canal. In this position, molding (the coning of the baby's head that makes the diameter smaller to more easily fit through the pelvis) happens more easily. Labor with an OA, LOA or LOT baby can be shorter and less painful than with other fetal positions.

Today, midwife Gail Tully adds body balancing to OFP and calls it Spinning Babies®

For much more information about optimal fetal positioning, including many positions and techniques not listed here please visit Gail Tully's website Spinning Babies® at www.spinningbabies.com. Gail has brilliantly identified 3 principals in helping to achieve and maintain good fetal positioning; I have used her techniques for many years with tremendous success and highly recommend them. Those three principals are Balance, Movement and Gravity. We will explore them more in the following pages.

FETAL POSITIONS

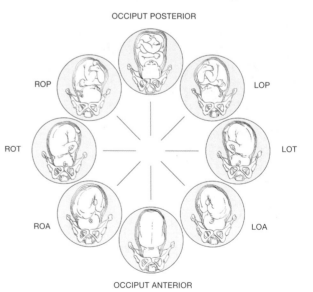

OCCIPUT POSTERIOR

ROP

LOP

ROT

LOT

ROA

LOA

OCCIPUT ANTERIOR

To establish and keep babies in an OA or LOA position, we use balancing positions along with movement and gravity.

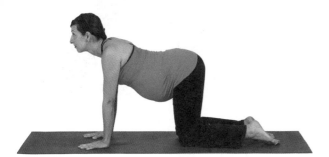
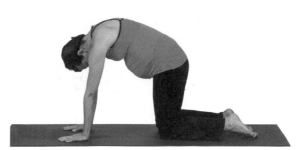

1

Leaning forward or being on your hands and knees doing pelvic tilts is effective in labor to help encourage optimal positioning, using the contractions to aid in turning babies.

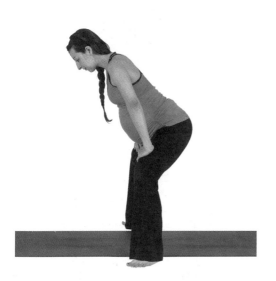
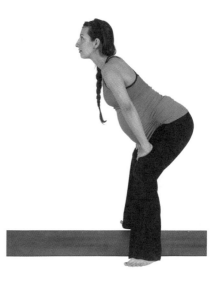

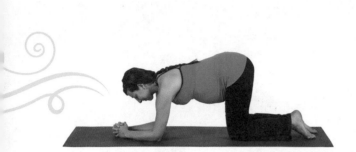

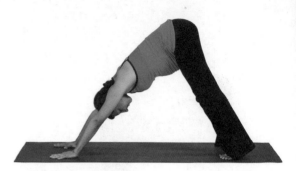

2

Keeping the womb symmetrical and stable, using movement and gravity as well as short inversions to relax the uterine ligaments. Inversions can also be helpful to make the pelvic floor more symmetrical.

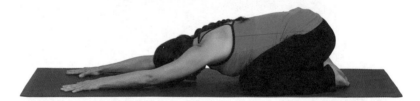

3

Keeping the pelvic floor in balance is another important aspect of balancing the womb. Child's pose and squats are helpful here.

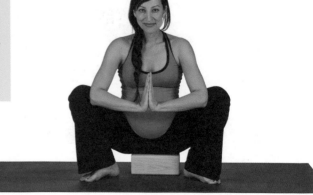

BREECH AND TRANSVERSE BABIES

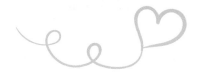

A breech baby is a baby who is presenting with the bottom down and head up. Technically any baby who is not in a head down position is considered "breech." including those who are lying sideways in the uterus (transverse). It is important to understand that just because a baby is in a breech position does not necessarily mean there is anything wrong. Many babies are born vaginally in a breech position all over the world every day. It used to be much more common for babies to be delivered with a breech presentation, but now many doctors are uncomfortable delivering breech babies and will automatically do a cesarean if a baby is breech. Since this is a leading cause of cesarean due to fetal positioning, let's explore some ways to help turn babies who are breech to get them into head-down positions."

POSITIONS AND TECHNIQUES FOR TURNING BREECH BABIES

The Breech Tilt **

I've found the best way to do this position is to place a yoga mat next to a wall, place a folded blanket under the mat right where the shoulders will be. Lay on the mat with the feet on the ground near the hips and touching the wall. Make sure the blanket is under the shoulders but not the neck; you want to have a space under the neck so that the spine doesn't get compressed. Place the feet flat on the wall and press into the wall with the feet lifting the hips up. Have someone then place 2 blocks with a folded blanket on top under the hips and straighten the legs on the wall. Optimally you want to have very little crease at the hips (imagine the shape your body would be in if you were lying on an ironing board that was propped up at an angle on a couch.) This will not be particularly comfortable for the mother, and baby might move around a bit. This can be further helped by using a cold compress wrapped in a towel, near the baby's head to encourage rotation away from the cold and possibly something warm near the pubic bone area. Visualization and talking to the baby is also very helpful to do during this inversion! I like to have women do a general relaxation and then have them talk to the baby, telling themselves and the baby that they are both safe and that it is ok to turn and that they are excited to see and hold the baby.

Forward Leaning Inversion **

This inversion is done for 30 seconds once daily, it can be done more gently by just elevating the knees on a bolster or 2 or the full inversion can be done with the knees on a sofa or heavy sturdy chair. The full forward inversion should be done SLOWLY and with assistance making sure there are no contraindications. The benefit of this pose comes from coming up afterwards, this movement brings the uterus into better alignment. The Forward Leaning Inversion was created by Dr. Carol Phillips, DC.

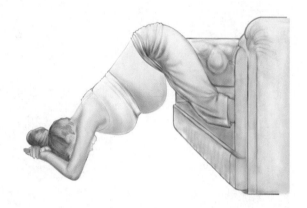

** Do not do inversions if you have any condition where inversions are contraindicated

Some conditions in which inversions are contraindicated are: High blood pressure; eye conditions such as glaucoma where pressure in the eyes needs to be avoided; heartburn; risk of stroke; unusually high levels of amniotic fluid; or if told not to invert by your doctor.

Pinky toe pressure point

The outside of the pinky toe is a pressure point that helps stimulate babies to turn from breech to a head-down position. Acupuncturists often use this point along with Moxibustion.

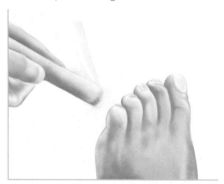

Moxibustion

External Cephalic Version

Many health care providers offer a technique called an external cephalic version. Done at around 37 weeks, this procedure is done by a healthcare provider physically turning the baby from the outside of the body.

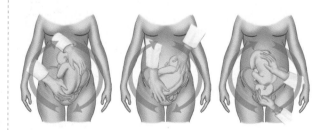

POSITIONS TO AVOID!

Just as important as knowing which positions are beneficial to fetal positioning is knowing which ones work against you and can lead to more physical discomfort and imbalance in the body.

SITTING

The way you sit and the amount of time you sit when you're pregnant can have a major impact on your body balance and comfort levels in pregnancy, ultimately affecting fetal positioning. Let's examine beneficial ways of sitting compared to positions that can encourage fetal malposition.

Sitting with an anterior tilt of the pelvis is most beneficial for ligament and muscular balance in the pregnant body. The reason is that the back of the baby's head and the back of the spine, are the heaviest parts of the body. So over time if a woman is constantly taking positions where she is leaning back or curving the lumbar spine, the baby will be encouraged by gravity to move into a position where the back of the head is against mom's spine. This position is the opposite of what is optimal for babies to come down through the pelvis. Starting labor in this position (called occipital posterior or OP) can make labor longer, sometimes leading to more back pain and discomfort. It is for this reason that we encourage so much forward leaning to help babies achieve good fetal positioning! You might be thinking, "That's great, but I have a job and need to sit down and drive a car; I can't live in a forward leaning position!" The idea is that when you sit, you sit in ways that promote good fetal positioning. Let's look at some easy tools to accomplish this goal, and explore the do's and don'ts of sitting in pregnancy.

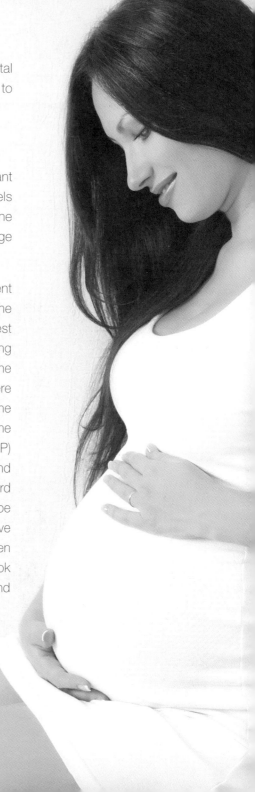

WAYS TO ACHIEVE GOOD
FETAL POSITIONING WHEN SITTING

- Sit on a ball

- Use a small towel roll under the crease where the thigh meets the buttocks and a small lumbar support pillow. Your sit bones should be pointing straight to the ground. This might seem like a lot of work, but you will be very happy to avoid some of the major discomforts that come with sitting improperly while pregnant.

- Embrace the squat position, if it isn't already part of your daily life. Getting comfortable with this position can help you so much in birthing. Squatting can create a much bigger opening of the bottom of the pelvis to accommodate the baby's head and shoulders. It is said that the squat can increase the bottom (inferior) opening of the pelvis by up to 30 percent in comparison to lying down on a bed and lifting the legs up to deliver the baby! (Don't worry; we will talk about this more later!)

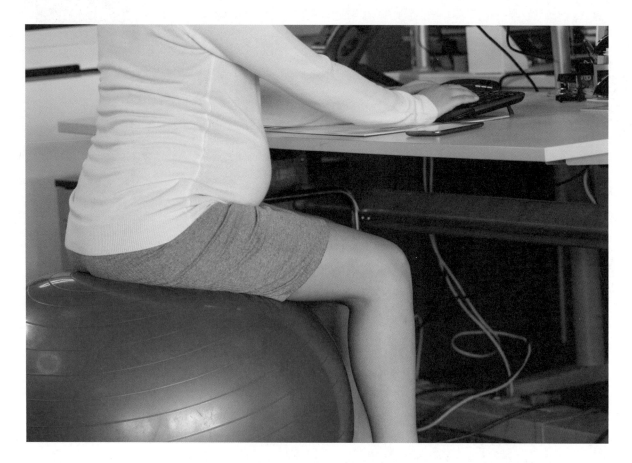

WHAT TO AVOID

Leaning back on soft couches or chairs for long periods of time, can cause the lumbar spine (lower back) to curve towards the ground. This rounding of the lower back, when done on a regular basis, can lead to lower back pain and does not encourage good fetal positioning. I have noticed an increase of babies in positions that were not conducive to birthing after the women were on bed rest for long periods of time. These women usually would spend time leaning back on pillows in bed or on the couch. It's a good idea to check out the latest research on bed rest to examine if you and your doctor think it is right for you. The American College of Obstetricians and Gynecologists (ACOG) has recently given the following recommendation "Don't routinely recommend activity restriction or bed rest during pregnancy for any indication. Bed rest or activity restriction has been commonly recommended for a variety of conditions in pregnancy, including multiple gestation, intrauterine growth restriction, preterm labor, premature rupture of membranes, vaginal bleeding, and hypertensive disorders in pregnancy. However, information to date does not show an improvement in birth outcome with the use of bed rest or activity restriction but does show an increase in loss of muscle conditioning and thromboembolic disease."[11]

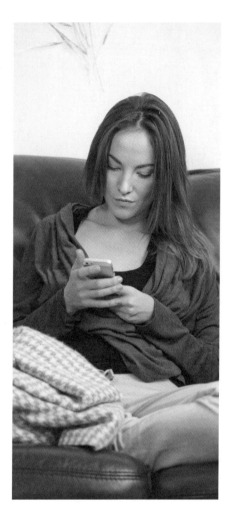

Don't sit too long!

Try to avoid sitting for more than about 20 minutes at one time. Unlike other ligaments in the body, the ligaments of the uterus have contractile tissue in them, similar to muscle tissue, that allows them to contract and lengthen. When you sit for long periods of time, some of the ligaments can shorten, pulling the uterus into a position that can cause discomfort for mom and less than optimal positioning for baby. This is one of the reasons that a woman will feel a pulling sensation or pain when standing after sitting for a long time.

Avoid soft chairs

Stay away from chairs that don't provide any lumbar support. I know those cozy soft chairs look so appealing when you're tired and just want to curl up and read a book, but they might create more discomfort in the long run and are not the best choice to encourage optimal fetal positioning.

ADDITIONAL WAYS TO ACHIEVE GOOD FETAL POSITIONING

Practice prenatal yoga

In the next chapter, you'll see a gentle sequence that you can use daily that will take about 15 minutes. This practice can help to balance the body and may relieve or prevent many of the common pregnancy discomforts. Make sure that you do only positions that feel good; you should never have any pain while doing these poses. Also make sure you have informed your doctor that you are doing prenatal yoga, in case there are any medical issues that might affect which pose you can or cannot do.

Meditation and visualization

This can encourage baby to move into an optimal position. Just 10 or 15 minutes a few times a week of positive visualization can be very helpful in easing stress and anxiety, and encouraging positive positioning. See Chapter 10 for suggestions.

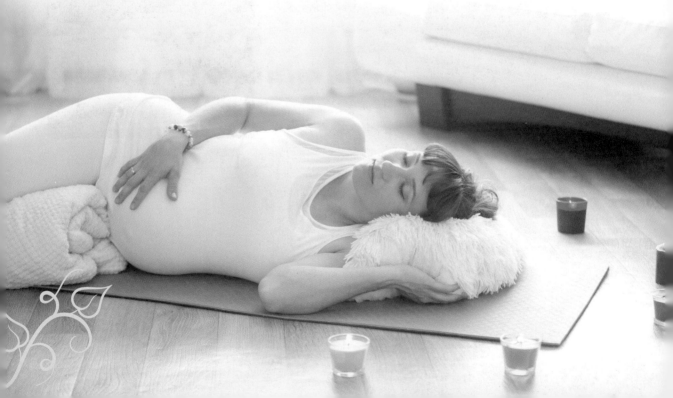

OTHER VERY USEFUL BALANCING TECHNIQUES YOU WILL FIND ON THE SPINNING BABIES WEBSITE THAT I HAVE HAD A LOT OF SUCCESS WITH ARE:

The Side Lying Release

This is a wonderful tool for pregnant women to use once or twice during late pregnancy. It's helpful for any pregnant woman but especially for those who are dancers, runners, Pilates practitioners, or who do any sport or activity which strengthens or can create tightness in the pelvic floor. The Side Lying Release is also great for those who have had a previous cesarean, breech or other mal-positioned baby, failure to progress in a previous labor, those who have pelvic, back or hip pain, a baby that is very high and not engaging after 38 weeks, or pain with intercourse

Rebozo Sifting

This is one of my all time favorite techniques. It's very comfortable and safe for most women. I have used this technique with hundreds of pregnant women with really favorable outcomes and very highly recommend it. Here are some things I have seen this technique work for: relaxing tight uterine ligaments; helping with lower back pain; helping babies find a good position in labor; and encouraging labor to resume if it slows down or stops.

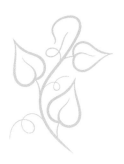

Spinning Babies, The Breech Tilt, Forward Leaning Inversion, Side Lying Release, Rebozo Sifting

Chapter 4

YOGA

EVERYWHERE YOU GO THESE DAYS PEOPLE ARE TALKING ABOUT THE BENEFITS OF PRENATAL YOGA. YOU'VE PROBABLY HEARD PEOPLE SAY, "YOGA IS THE BEST THING YOU CAN DO WHEN YOU'RE PREGNANT!" AND WONDERED WHY YOGA IS GETTING ALL OF THIS INTERNATIONAL ATTENTION.

The obvious reasons have to do with the impact of yoga on calming the mind and reducing stress as well as increasing physical and mental strength and flexibility. All of these are great reasons to continue a yoga practice while pregnant or to begin a yoga practice during pregnancy. There is, however, an important reason that is talked about less frequently that has benefits that can affect your pregnancy as well as your labor, delivery and postpartum recovery. It is yoga's role in helping to achieve and maintain optimal fetal positioning that we've just discussed in the previous chapter.

During pregnancy, women experience dramatic physical, emotional, and mental transformations in which they have an amazing opportunity to connect for a short time with another human being in an incredibly intimate way. The life inside them is continually growing and changing.

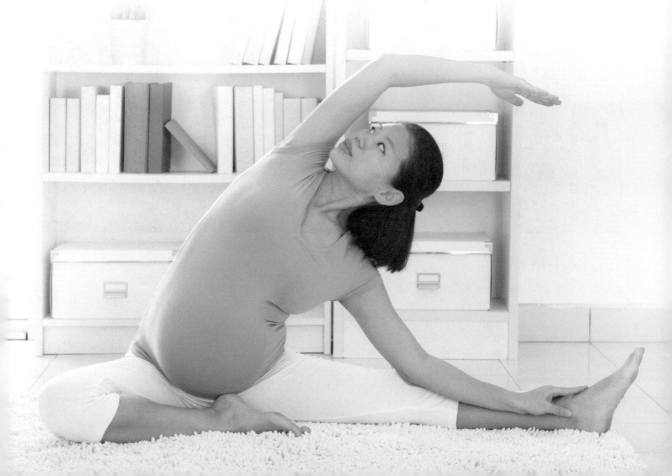

The movement of the woman's breath and body are enabling, encouraging and creating that growth, as it feeds the life inside her. Vinyasa yoga is the linking of body movement and breath, enabling the continuous flow of energy through the body. The movement of body and breath are one, connected, continuously flowing and synchronized. When a practitioner learns to link breath and movement, they create an energy that powerfully connects them to their own being. Bringing this experience of connectedness to pregnant women in a physical, tangible way is the intention of Prenatal Vinyasa Yoga. Prenatal yoga is so powerful because it continuously reminds a woman that even as her muscles are being challenged, she can keep her breath and energy moving through her body, releasing the parts of her body that are not working and allowing them to relax as she builds strength and endurance.

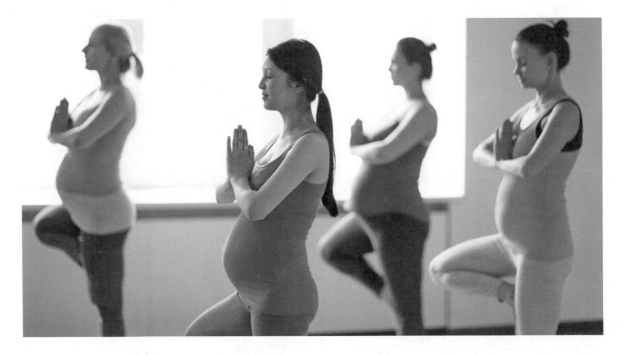

This breath and movement connection becomes pivotal in childbirth because the tendency in intense fear or pain is to freeze, hold the breath, tense up all muscles, even those that aren't working, and stop any forward movement. When a woman connects her breath and body in labor, it is an empowering and beautiful thing. Learning Vinyasa Yoga in pregnancy gives women the ability to feel continuous energy movement in labor and to embrace that movement, linking it to her breath and allowing it to grow, creating an ecstatic, empowering birth experience. The focus and connection with the breath allows a woman to tap into the rhythm of her body and work with it instead of fighting it.

Many women who regularly practice prenatal yoga have faster and less painful birth experiences than those who don't do this. Of course, there are many exceptions and circumstances that increase length and intensity of labor, but the yoga correlation is too great to ignore or write off as just coincidence. I was thrilled when a study from Thailand aligned with my own observations and confirmed my theory. The Thailand study found women who did prenatal yoga experienced more comfort during pregnancy, shorter and more manageable births with less pain, fewer medical interventions and speedier postpartum recoveries. I believe there are several reasons for the outcomes observed in Thailand.

1. Yoga can increase lung capacity allowing the woman to take deeper and longer breaths, which bring oxygen to the baby and mom, making contractions feel shorter and more manageable. A woman in a yoga class is encouraged not to hold her breath or tense up, but to breathe deeply and directly into the tension. When a woman is tense, the contractions can feel much more intense.

2. Women who do prenatal yoga tend to have more stamina (especially when practicing styles such as Prenatal Vinyasa Yoga which builds strength and flexibility while staying focused on the breath and on releasing tension). Therefore they can go a longer time without pain medication. In my experience, when women get pain medication, it tends to slow down labor.

3. Prenatal yoga releases endorphins or "feel good" hormones that a woman becomes accustomed to feeling while practicing yoga. These same hormones are released during labor and are much more identifiable to women who have been practicing yoga.

4. Practicing relaxation at the end of class helps women to become familiar with what their bodies feel like when they are comfortable and free of tension. It also gives them a practice of staying in the moment and focused.

The practice of prenatal yoga provides women with many physical and mental advantages when it comes time for them to give birth, but prenatal yoga works best for women when it is practiced often. Here is a 15- minute sequence you can do every day to help achieve some of the amazing benefits that prepare your body, mind, and spirit for pregnancy, birth and beyond. I encourage you to do this practice daily and, if possible, to integrate the longer 60-minute practice I've included a few times a week!

THE DOLPHIN METHOD
15-MINUTE PRACTICE

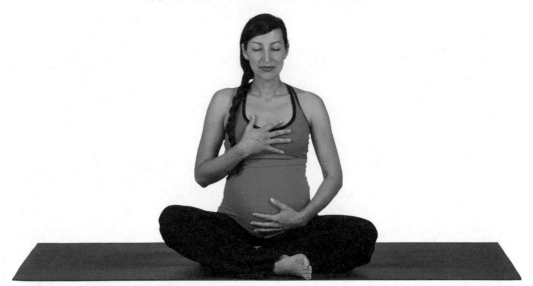

SEATED HAND ON HEART

- Take a couple of deep breaths.
- Check in with your body.
- Respect where your body is today, remember that your body is your baby's home until she is born so be kind to it.
- Allow for days when your body needs more rest or a more gentle practice.
- And most of all listen to the signs your body gives you. Iif you have discomfort or pain, back off and rest.
- Begin Ujjayi breath by breathing in and out through the nose, slightly constricting the back of the throat (inhale and exhale) which makes a soft sound, like the ocean waves. On the exhale, imagine hugging your baby in, towards the spine. Use this breath throughout the practice, especially in forward-leaning positions, to support the stomach muscles.
- If your breath becomes uneven or labored reduce the intensity of your practice until it evens out.
- Introduce the concepts of practicing with intention and attention.

Modifications:

- Sitting on the knees or in Hero pose sitting on a block, or elevate the hips in a cross-legged position.

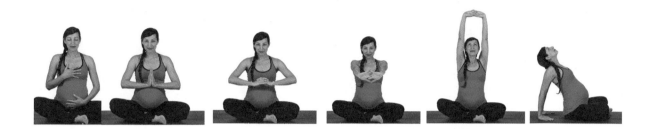

Seated hands on heart, hands in prayer, interlace fingers reach up, hands behind back lift chest.

- Lengthen spine as you reach arms overhead.
- Keeping spine long, bring arms behind the back resting on the hands reaching the chest forward and up
- Release head back.

Modifications:

- If it doesn't feel good to bring the head back, just lengthen the neck and look up.

Side Stretch

- Lengthen spine as you reach arms overhead.
- Keeping spine long bring one arm down at a time and lengthen up and over to the opposite side with the other arm.

Modifications:

- Arm can stay straight up if it is uncomfortable to reach up and over.

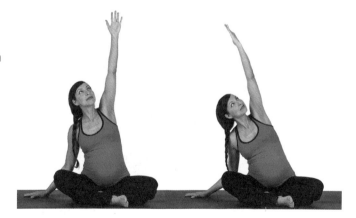

Cat/Cow (Marjaryasana)

- Make sure the hands are directly under the shoulders.
- Knees hip-width apart, directly under the hips.
- Try not to sway the back as you inhale.
- As you exhale, press the hands into the mat to exaggerate the roundness of the back, and drop the head down. Gently hug baby into the spine.
- This is a pose that should be done every day.
- If your baby is in an uncomfortable position, it can help to turn your baby into a position which is more comfortable for you.
- This also can help to turn your baby, in labor, into a position which is more comfortable for you and more conducive for baby to be birthed.
- For Cat/Cow Circles, bring hands forward and wider, and widen knees.

Modifications:

- Alternate leg/arm lift

Carpal Tunnel variations:

- Hands in fists
- Wedge
- Rolled up mat

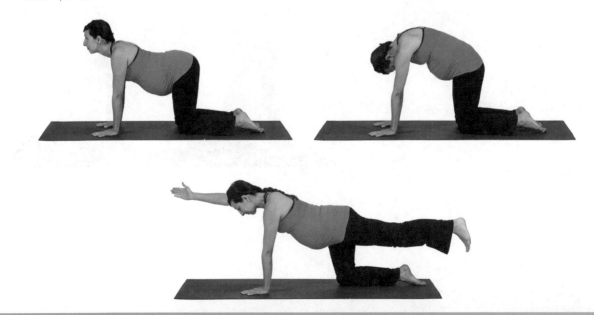

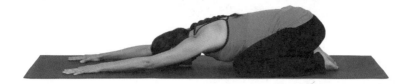

CHILD'S POSE (BALASANA)

• Separate knees, sit down on heels, bring forehead to ground, reach arms out in front.

Modifications:

• Place block or bolster under head if needed.

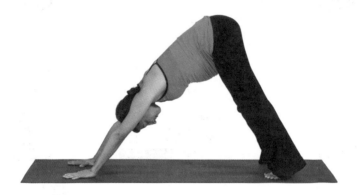

DOWNWARD FACING DOG (ADHO MUKHA SVANASANA)

• From hands and knees, curl toes under lift hips.
• Feet hip-width apart or more to create space for baby.

Modifications:

• If downward dog is uncomfortable or counter indicated move into child's pose instead.

** Do not do inversions if you have any condition where inversions are contraindicated

Some conditions in which inversions are contraindicated are: High blood pressure; eye conditions such as glaucoma where pressure in the eyes needs to be avoided; heartburn; risk of stroke; unusually high levels of amniotic fluid; or if told not to invert by your doctor.

Soft Form Vinyasa Flow

1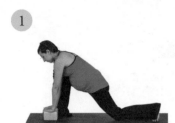

Bring the right foot forward and knee down.

Modification:
Different block heights

2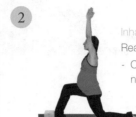

Inhale
Reach the arms up
- One hand can come to thigh if needed.

3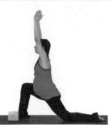

Exhale
Lunge forward
- Make sure knee doesn't go past the toes and the front foot stays flat on the floor.
- Make sure the lunge isn't too deep by hugging baby into the spine during exhalation.

4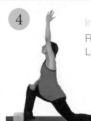

Inhale
Right elbow on right thigh
Left arm reaches up.

5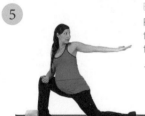

Exhale
Reach arm open to the back of the room.
- Palm up

6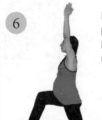

Inhale
Lengthen both arms up.

7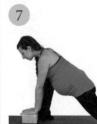

Exhale
Release hands back to the inside of the right foot.
- Bring right knee back to the floor.

8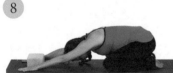

Inhale
All fours
Exhale
Child's pose

9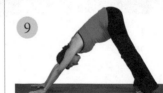

Exhale
Downward dog
1 to 3 breaths

10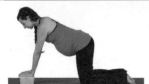

Exhale
Release knees down back to all fours.
Inhale
Bring the thumbs together with the fingers spread out wide - hands come forward slightly and can be on a block or on the ground.

11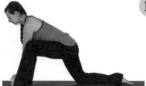

Exhale
Bring the left foot to the outside of the left hand.

12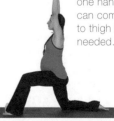

Inhale
Reach the arms up - one hand can come to thigh if needed.

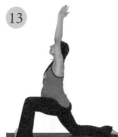

13 Exhale

Lunge forward

- Make sure knee doesn't go past the toes and the front foot stays flat on the floor.
- Make sure the lunge isn't too deep by hugging baby into the spine during exhalation.

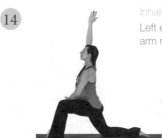

14 Inhale

Left elbow on left thigh right arm reaches up .

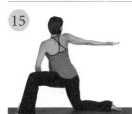

15 Exhale

Reach arm open to the back of the room palm up.

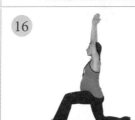

16 Inhale

Lengthen both arms up.

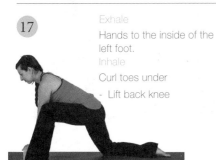

17 Exhale

Hands to the inside of the left foot.
Inhale
Curl toes under
- Lift back knee

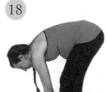

18 Exhale

Step right foot forward.
Inhale
Lengthen spine

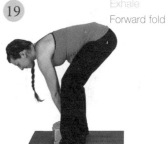

19 Exhale

Forward fold

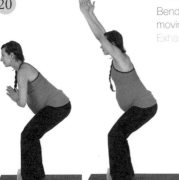

20 Inhale

Bend knees deeply moving into chair pose.
Exhale

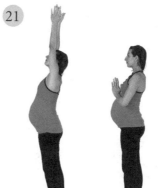

21 Inhale

To standing

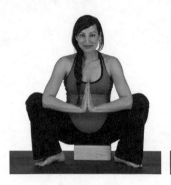 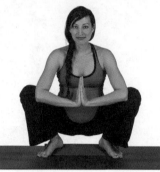

SQUAT

(make sure both heels are on the floor or use a modification)

Modifications:

- Bolster or Block
- Wedge or Blanket under the heels

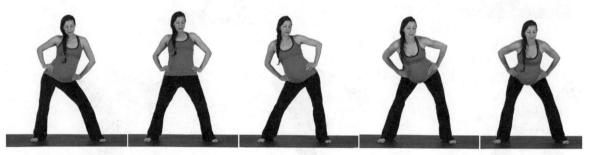

HIP CIRCLES

(feet wide, knees bent)

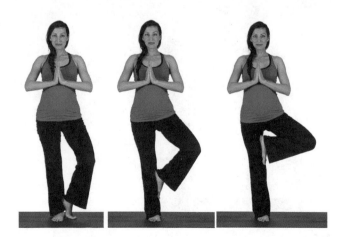

TREE POSE

Modifications:

- Foot can be on the ground, ankle, calf, or thigh.
- Don't put foot on the knee.
- Arms can be in prayer or up.

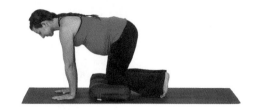

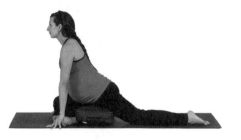

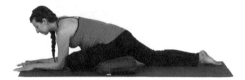

Pigeon

Over a rolled up blanket or bolster. Or double pigeon
(1 minute each side)

- Start with knees on a rolled up blanket.
- Hands forward
- Right leg forward and turned out
- Slide back so both hips are supported evenly
- Hips square to the ground
- Double pigeon (Stack shins, flex feet)

Modifications:

- Can be done from downward dog if advanced
- Can be done on a bolster if the blanket is too low
- Double Pigeon (block under the knee if needed)

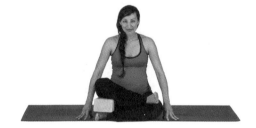

Side Lunge

- Line up heel with knee.
- Walk hands forward and widen them.
- Turn toes to face the side of the room.
- Lunge to the side then circles if comfortable.

Modifications:

- Foot can move forward or back to make it more comfortable

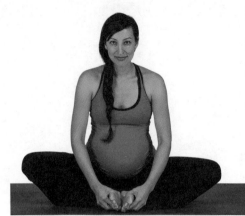

BOUND ANGLE

Modifications:

• If baby is breech and Mom is past 34-35 weeks, cross legs instead.

• Place blocks or blankets under the knees if needed.

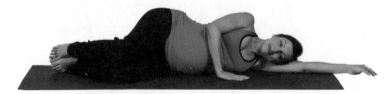

SIDE-RECLINING LEG LIFT

Optional:

• Quad stretch

• Reaching back for the foot

• Thigh parallel to the ground

• Move leg back until the stretch is felt at the front of the thigh.

• Happy baby in between sides

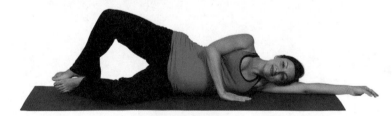

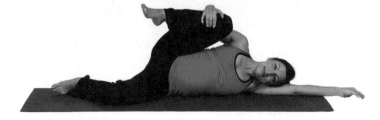

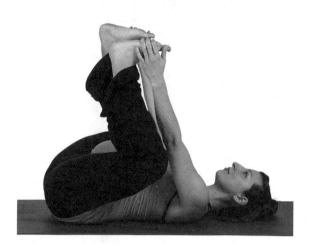

HAPPY BABY POSE

Rock side to side

FINAL RELAXATION
RECLINING BOUND ANGLE

Use a rolled up blanket or a block under each thigh to support the hips.

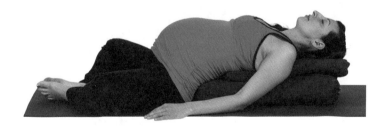

 For more yoga sequences, visit the website

Chapter 5

AVOID
INDUCTION

If a woman's labor doesn't start on its own, a medical practitioner may decide to help her labor get started. This is referred to as labor induction. Labor induction is done using several different techniques to prepare and dilate the cervix. (See chart below.) The purpose of these techniques is typically to soften or ripen the cervix and bring on contractions. Research shows that, in the US, around one in five births starts with an induction. Inductions are most commonly done if the doctor or midwife feels it is safer for mom and/or baby for the baby to be delivered sooner rather than waiting for nature to take its course.

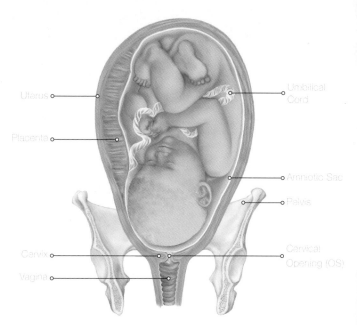

In order to understand induction, it is important to become familiar with some terms and the basic anatomy of pregnancy and childbirth. Take a look at this chart below to familiarize yourself with the parts of the body we will discuss when we talk about induction.

CERVICAL DILATION & EFFACEMENT

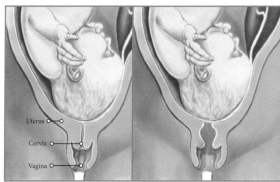

Cervix is not effaced or dilated.

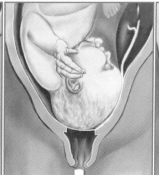

Cervix is dilated to 1cm.

Cervix is is fully effaced and dilated to 5cm.

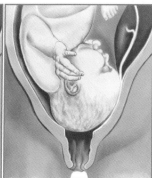

Cervix is fully dilated to 10cm.

MOST COMMON REASONS FOR INDUCTION

Due date

A woman's due date is typically calculated to be 40 weeks from the first day of her last menstrual period. It is common to get an ultrasound in the first trimester of pregnancy to confirm the due date and viability of the pregnancy. Ultrasounds done in the first trimester are more accurate in determining fetal age than ultrasounds done in subsequent trimesters. This is important to know because sometimes due dates will get changed based on second- or third-trimester ultrasounds, leading to women being induced unnecessarily.

Many hospitals and doctors follow a protocol of not allowing women to go more than one to two weeks past the due date or 40th week.[12] As the fetus and placenta mature, the placenta eventually starts to calcify and therefore becomes less effective at bringing essential nutrients and oxygen to the baby. At home births, there is often more flexibility about using induction when a woman's due date has passed. Women have been known to go successfully three or more weeks past their due dates without intervention.

Water breaking

Inductions are also done when a woman's water breaks and she is not having contractions. The baby is protected inside of a sealed sac of amniotic fluid. Most of the time, a woman's water breaks some time during her labor. About 15 percent of the time, water breaks before labor begins. Typically when this happens, labor will begin within about 24 hours. Depending on the doctor, situation, or hospital policy, doctors will induce labor if contractions don't begin within six to 24 hours after the water breaks. There are doctors who will allow women to wait longer than 24 hours, but that is less common. At home births, midwives have more flexibility and, depending on the situation, may allow women whose waters have broken to wait until contractions begin on their own, even if this takes several days.

Q Ultrasounds, water breaks

Amniotic fluid

If a woman gets an ultrasound late in pregnancy and her levels of amniotic fluid are considered abnormal, either too low (oligohydramnios) or too high (polyhydramnios), this could lead to a doctor's decision to induce. There are several possible causes for low or high levels of amniotic fluid, some of which are dangerous and some of which are not. It is always best to do some research and get a second opinion if these diagnoses are made.

Large Baby

One of the most common reasons for induction in many countries is when a woman gets a diagnosis of having a large baby and/or a small pelvis. As the pregnancy progresses past the due date, a baby's increasing size gives rise to concern that the baby might not fit as easily through the mom's pelvis. This is a common issue when a woman has been diagnosed with gestational diabetes. Having a very large baby can increase the risk of the baby getting juvenile diabetes, shoulder distocia, or birth trauma.

For women who do not have gestational diabetes, there are a couple of things to consider if your doctor is contemplating induction because he or she is concerned that your baby is going to be too big to deliver vaginally. The first factor is that the baby's weight is usually determined by an ultrasound that can be inaccurate by up to pound and a half in either direction! Therefore, many moms who are induced for having large babies in fact deliver normal-size babies.

The second factor to consider is that the only way to determine if a pelvis can accommodate the baby is to have an x-ray of the pelvis. Measuring the pelvis from the outside will not give you an accurate determination. We also need to consider that a woman's body is made to be able to give birth vaginally! A woman's pelvis has greater mobility during pregnancy to allow it to open up more (especially when a woman is not lying in bed). If the baby is in a good position in the pelvis, the diameter of the head will get much smaller due to the molding of the skull, creating a cone shape that allows the baby to fit through a smaller area.

gestational diabetes, shoulder distocia

Health concerns of mom or baby

There are certain health conditions that sometimes prompt doctors or midwives to induce labor. If a woman's blood pressure is too high or she has preeclampsia, gestational diabetes, heart disease, an infection, or if there is bleeding during pregnancy for any number of reasons that make her "high risk," induction may be recommended.

Maternal Request

Let's face it, many women get tired of being pregnant by the time their due date comes around. Swollen ankles, frequent urination, sleep interruption, and anxiety about when the baby will arrive are all factors that go into a woman's choice to be induced. Unfortunately, most women do not understand that the process of induction can be long, tiring, and filled with medical interventions that ultimately can increase the chance of her having a cesarean.

My best advice for women who are considering induction for these reasons is to cherish these last days or weeks of pregnancy as a time of special union with your baby. Although it can be difficult, pregnancy brings a closeness you will forever treasure. Remember that pregnancy is a journey that takes us to the brink of our fears and discomfort so that we can emerge into motherhood with strength and confidence. As with many journeys, the end feels impossibly difficult, and we just want it to be over. The last days of pregnancy, however, are a pivotal part of the journey, because it is in this time that we are shown our own depth and potential.

I recommend focusing on the things that feel good for your body at this time. Get into water, a bath or a pool, and notice how good it feels to float. Take this time for intimacy with your partner. Have a date and enjoy each other's company. Embrace this time when you are encouraged to take care of yourself, as your focus will soon turn to taking care of someone else.

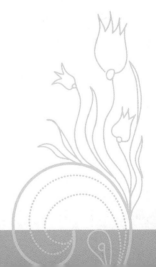

preeclampsia

WHAT IS INDUCTION AND HOW IS IT DONE?

There are several different ways to induce labor. While natural induction techniques can usually be done outside of the hospital, medical induction is done at a hospital or birthing facility.

Medical induction

The kind of medical induction a woman is given depends upon the state of her body at the time of induction. The first thing a doctor will do is to check her cervix and assess its ripeness to determine which induction techniques are most appropriate.

Preparing the cervix

If her cervix has not started to efface or dilate, it is considered unripe and not ready for labor. In this case, hormones or mechanical methods to ripen the cervix will be used. Occasionally, this is enough to get labor going without further intervention.

The most common substances used to help ripen the cervix are hormone-like substances called prostaglandins that are usually inserted into the vagina and onto the cervix via a suppository. These suppositories are left in for a number of hours and can be taken out when the cervix is ripened or if labor begins. Many times women will experience mild contractions while the prostaglandins are taking effect. Once the cervix has ripened, other hormones can be administered to initiate contractions and bring on labor.

Another method of preparing the cervix uses a Foley Catheter inflated with water to stretch out the cervix. A balloon of water is placed inside the cervix, and when the cervix dilates to about four centimeters, the balloon falls out. This method can only be used when some cervical dilation has already occurred.

prostaglandin, Foley Catheter

Another mechanical method for preparing the cervix is called stripping or sweeping the membrane. During this method, the health-care provider uses her fingers inserted into the cervix to gently separate the bag of water (amniotic sac) from the side of the uterus by sweeping her fingers back and forth. This method can only be used when the cervix has some opening.

Starting Contractions

Once ripe enough, the cervix opens up in a process called dilation. The cervix dilates in response to uterine contractions. If contractions are not strong enough, the cervix will not open.

Contractions are brought on when a woman's body releases the hormone oxytocin. The release of oxytocin during labor causes contractions that help move the baby down, allowing the pressure of the baby's head to stimulate cervical opening. These contractions also help expel the placenta and keep a woman from bleeding too much after her baby and placenta have been birthed.

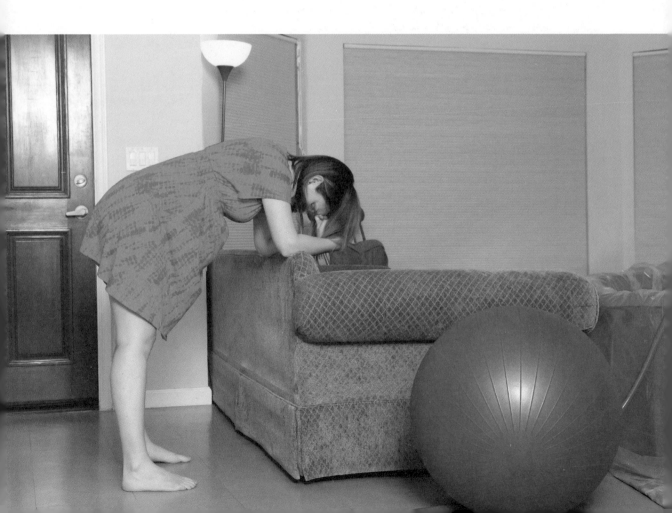

When a woman is medically induced, she is given a synthetic form of oxytocin called Pitocin. Most of the time, Pitocin brings on uterine contractions. Because Pitocin is a synthetic form of oxytocin, sometimes women's bodies don't respond to it in the same way that they respond to their own bodies' oxytocin. Problems can range from contractions being too intense and stressing out the baby to the mother's body not recognizing the hormone and contractions not starting at all.

Occasionally, doctors will break the bag of water in order to start contractions. This will bring the baby's head down onto the cervix, and the pressure of the baby's head will stimulate cervical change. This method has both benefits and disadvantages. Once the water is broken, doctors like to see the baby delivered within a short period of time to minimize the likelihood of infection. If contractions don't begin soon after breaking the water, further medical interventions are likely. It's important to note that the likelihood of infection increases the more vaginal exams are done, so most protocols include having no more than three vaginal exams done after the water has broken and before the delivery of the baby. At home births, many midwives will forego vaginal exams entirely to decrease the chance of infection.

If the baby is not in a good position when the water is broken, the decrease in amniotic fluid makes it harder for a baby to achieve optimal position, therefore increasing the chances the baby will get "stuck" in a position that does not allow him or her to easily move through the pelvis. To compound this, sometimes when the water is broken, doctors will insist that a woman stay in bed. This position makes it even more difficult for babies to attain optimal position.

The reason that doctors sometimes insist on keeping the woman in bed after the water has broken is that they are afraid of the umbilical cord being pushed under the baby's head and through the cervix. This is called cord prolapse and is very dangerous because when the cord gets pinched between the head and the cervix, it cuts off oxygen to the baby. Many doctors now recognize that once the water has broken and the head comes down onto the cervix, there is very little chance that the cord will slip down under the baby's head if a woman is upright and moving around, because gravity is keeping the baby's head firmly against the cervix.

oxytocin, Pitocin

RISKS OF MEDICAL INDUCTIONS

While induction is generally safe, it carries some risks that vary according to the methods used and the individual situation. As we discussed earlier, Pitocin can sometimes over-stimulate the uterus, meaning the contractions come too frequently or are abnormally long and strong. This in turn can stress the baby. In rare cases, Pitocin can also cause placental abruption or even uterine rupture, although ruptures are extremely rare in women who have never had a C-section or other uterine surgery. Labor induction can take a long time, especially if you are starting with an unripe cervix. Because women must be at the hospital continuously throughout an induction, they can get very fatigued before the hard part of labor even begins. This can lead to the mother becoming emotionally distressed or disappointed and requesting early pain medication or even a cesarean.

USE YOUR B.R.A.I.N.

Here is a wonderful formula for assessing your options when faced with a healthcare provider, nurse, doctor or midwife who is recommending an intervention. Using this formula will help you understand why you need the intervention or might open up a dialogue about it that will ultimately lead to avoiding unnecessary interventions.

THE ACRONYM B.R.A.I.N. STANDS FOR:

BENEFITS

What are the benefits of this procedure? How will this help my labor, my baby, or me?

RISKS

What are the risks of this procedure? How might this negatively affect my labor, my baby, or me?

ALTERNATIVES

Are there alternatives to this procedure? What are my other options?

INTUITION

What is my gut feeling about this?

NEED TIME

What if I choose to do nothing for now, what are the implications? Can I delay this procedure and take some time to think about it and discuss it with my partner?

NATURAL METHODS OF INDUCTION

Knowing the potential risks and downsides of medical induction, it is worth considering some natural induction techniques before going down the medical route. Make sure that you talk to your health-care provider before using any of the natural induction techniques discussed in this book.

Here are some of the most common and, in my experience, most successful natural techniques:

Acupuncture

By far my favorite natural induction technique is acupuncture. Please note that it is important to find a practitioner who is experienced in working with pregnant women.

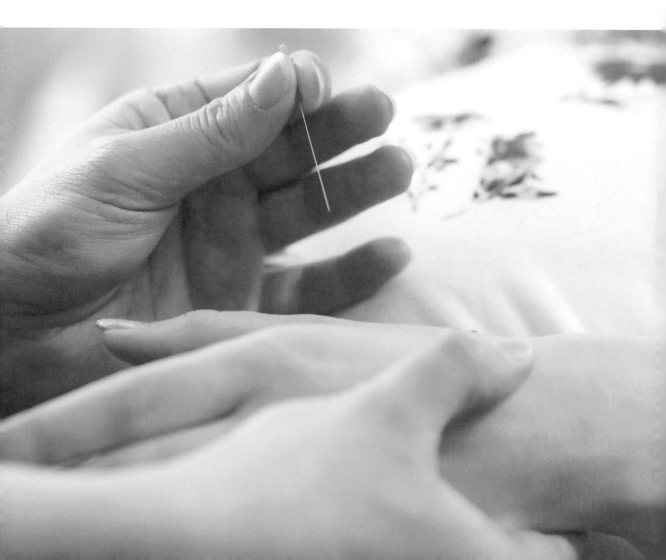

Acupressure

This is one of the simplest techniques that a mother or her partner can do. There are numerous acupressure points that can help bring on labor, if the body and the baby are ready.

Chiropractic adjustment

This can be very effective to align the body because it allows the baby to move down into the pelvis, which then stimulates labor if the mom's body and baby are ready for this process to begin.

Ingesting Castor Oil

Ingesting castor oil for induction is a little bit controversial and should be discussed with your healthcare provider before choosing this method. Taking small amounts (1 tablespoon) of castor oil mixed with juice every few hours seems to work well for most women without having a lot of negative side effects.[13] It is important to make sure you are using the proper kind of castor oil, as there are several different kinds. Some are topical while others are for internal use. Be sure anything you take is approved for internal use.

Intercourse

There is a saying in the childbirth industry: "The energy that gets the baby in, gets the baby out." Intercourse can be effective in several different ways. The first is that semen has prostaglandins in it that, if the cervix is ready, will help ripen it. Secondly, when a woman enjoys intercourse and the closeness associated with it, her body releases oxytocin, the same hormone that is needed to contract the uterus. This is especially effective if her nipples get stimulated.

Homeopathic remedies and herbs

If you want to use herbs, it's important to do so under the care of a licensed herbalist who has experience working with labor induction. These herbs can be very dangerous if taken in improper amounts but can be effective if used properly. Homeopathic remedies are popular, gentle and need to be taken with the advice of a trained homeopath, midwife and/or doctor.

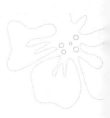

See website for list of acupressure points

Eating dates

There was a 2011 study conducted and published in the Journal of Obstetrics and Gynecology[14] comparing women who consumed six dates per day in the last four weeks of pregnancy and those who didn't. "It is concluded that the consumption of date fruit in the last four weeks before labour significantly reduced the need for induction and augmentation of labour, and produced a more favorable, but non significant, delivery outcome… Spontaneous labour occurred in 96% of

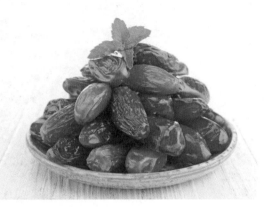

those who consumed dates, compared to 79% women in the non-date fruit consumers…Use of prostin/oxytocin was significantly lower in women who consumed dates (28%) compared with the non date fruit consumers (47%)."

Other

Here are some other commonly discussed natural folk traditions. You can choose to try them if you'd like, though there is not necessarily scientific evidence that they work.

- Eating spicy food
- Exercise
- Red raspberry leaf tea
- Guided relaxation
- Eating pineapple
- Induction massage

Chapter 6

CREATE YOUR ENVIRONMENT

THROUGHOUT NATURE, WE SEE EXAMPLES OF THE IMPORTANCE OF FEELING SAFE WHILE DELIVERING A BABY. IF AN ANIMAL IN THE WILD IS IN LABOR AND SENSES A THREAT, ITS LABOR WILL STOP AND NOT RESUME UNTIL THE ANIMAL FEELS SAFE.

Susan Graven, a midwife friend of mine, relayed a perfect example of the importance of feeling safe during the birthing process. In 1989 in California, there was a large earthquake. During that time, the labor and delivery floor of the hospital was full of women in varying stages of labor. When the earthquake hit, the lights went out, the building shook and everyone was afraid for their lives. When this occurred, labor stopped for every woman on that floor, and their labors did not resume until the lights went back on and they felt safe again.

Most women in the U.S. and those in major cities throughout the world deliver their babies in hospitals. What many people don't think about is that for most people, hospitals do not feel particularly safe. We go to hospitals when something is wrong or when someone is sick, so for many women just the act of stepping into the hospital creates an unsafe feeling or a sense of unease.

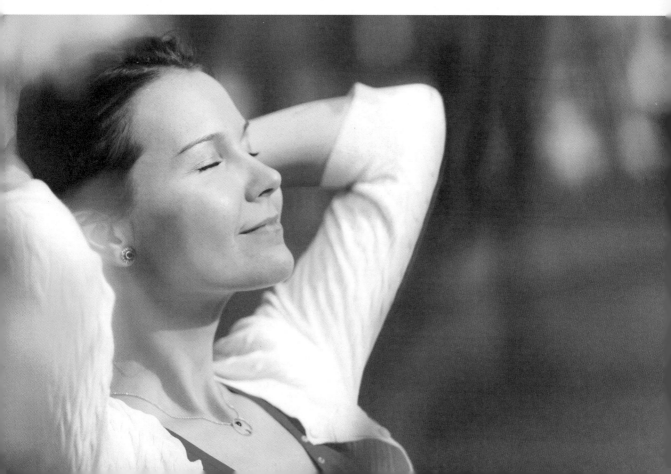

Once you get into your room at the hospital, that feeling often does not get any better. The hospital room is full of electronic equipment, always on the lookout for something wrong. The protocols followed by nurses and doctors tell them to evaluate problems and pain levels. The bright lights and constant observation and assessment of progress can and very often does create a heightened state of stress. The hormonal responses brought on by this stress increase a woman's adrenaline and cortisol levels (these are stress hormones), working against her natural endorphins, beta-endorphins and oxytocin, which help her labor progress and decrease pain levels.

Many midwives have observed that women prefer to give birth in a dark, quiet, undisturbed atmosphere. The same atmosphere in which a woman would want to make love is said to be the most conducive for birthing. This has been demonstrated time and time again in my personal experience of being with women as a doula for hundreds of births and in many documented accounts by authorities such as Ina May Gaskin, Penny Simkin, Debora Pascali-Bonaro, as well as many of my friends who are midwives, obstetricians, or doulas.

You don't need to feel resigned to the fact that if you have a hospital birth, you won't feel safe. You have much more control over the environment of your birth than you may think. With a little preparation and forethought, there are ways that you can make even the most basic hospital atmosphere feel safe and help your mind and body enjoy the birth of your baby.

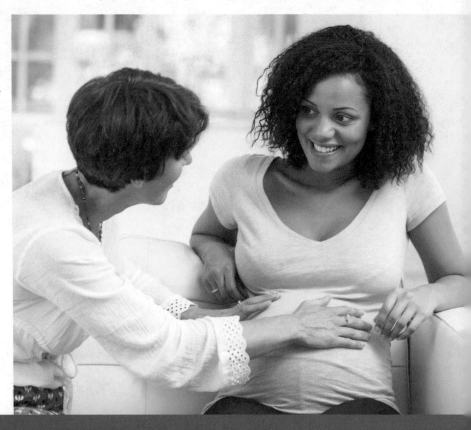

OPTIMIZING YOUR EXTERNAL ENVIRONMENT

One of the things that you can do to make the atmosphere of your birthing environment in a hospital feel safe is to bring things from home that will make the room feel less cold and medical. Things that you connect to - photos, special objects, even your own pillow and robe - can create a sense of comfort and well-being. Here are some ideas of things that could facilitate this safe feeling.

Feeling safe at the hospital

If a woman already has a fear of hospitals, just being there can make her feel insecure. I encourage women who know that they have this fear to go to the hospital sometime during their pregnancy, stand outside and think about this being the place where they are going to meet and hold their baby for the first time; then walk into the hospital holding that thought, creating new positive associations so that when she arrives in labor, she is able to walk into the hospital with less fear.

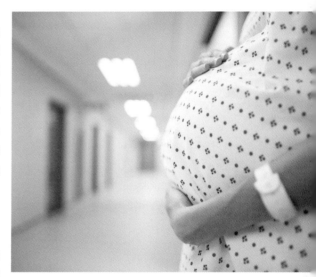

Scents, aromatherapy

The best way to use aromatherapy is to put the scent on a wet washcloth, not actually on your body, so that the scent can be taken away at any time if it becomes overwhelming or unpleasant.

Slippers, robe, and pillow

Make sure that you bring items that can get a little messy and can be washed or thrown away.

Lighting

Most hospital rooms have stark, bright lighting that is necessary in circumstances when doctors need to be able to perform certain tasks. However, this lighting is not optimal for laboring women. Women tend to prefer a cave-like atmosphere for birthing. Animals have similar instincts; you would never see an animal go into the center of a bright room to give birth. Luckily, during most of your labor, brightness of lighting can be controlled either by turning the lights down or by turning some of the lights off. Candlelight would be optimal, but you can't have actual flame in the hospital because of all the oxygen that's used there, so battery-operated candles are your next best option. Turn the lights down, and notice the calming effect changing the light in the room will have on your body's ability to relax, open up and give birth.

Sound

Hospitals are full of sounds that keep the nervous system on high alert and remind you of all the things that can possibly go wrong with birth. Some of the noises regularly found in a labor and delivery hospital room are fetal heart rate monitors, sounds from other women giving birth, and other medical equipment being used. Some hospital noises may contribute to a woman feeling unsafe in her environment and feeling as though she is a sick patient in a hospital when, in reality, she is not sick at all; she is giving birth to her baby. It may be a good idea to help a birthing woman regulate the noise in her room. Fetal heart rate monitors, for example, can be continuously on from the moment you get into the hospital. Some people find this sound comforting, while others hear the sounds and feel as though there is a constant threat of medical crisis. Fetal heart rate monitors have volume controls and can easily be turned down if requested. If they are contributing to anxiety, consider asking for intermittent monitoring and low volume.

Music is a great way to mask or de-emphasize these sounds and is a powerful way to change the mood of a room. I encourage all of my birthing mamas to create a playlist or two for their labor. Think about how music affects you on a regular basis. When you hear a song that you absolutely love come on the radio, you feel warm inside and happy. We have physical responses to music that can promote the feel-good hormones that are responsible for decreasing the pain of labor. If you like your music loud, bring headphones. Make sure your playlist includes music that can lift you up when you get tired or relax you when you get stressed. You also might want to include a guided visualization or recorded meditation that you enjoy doing.

Photos

Surround yourself with pictures that inspire you, bring you joy, and make you feel good. It could be pictures of nature or of loved ones whose energy is with you, reminding you that you're not alone and that you're loved.

People

Be aware of who you choose to have in the room with you during labor. Make sure that anyone you invite into the room is giving you energy and support at all times. We sometimes don't realize the effect that other people have on our physical and emotional state simply by their mere presence. I've talked to many obstetricians, midwives and doulas who agree that when there is even one person in a room with a birthing woman who is experiencing fatigue, burn out, or negative feelings about the experience, the effect on the birthing woman is evident. The effects range from her feeling greater fatigue to her labor slowing down or stopping due to her feeling unsafe. One technique for creating a supportive and safe atmosphere is to make sure that we arrange for positive support around us at all times. This could be a partner, friend or parent whom you trust, who makes you feel good when you are around them even if they have no experience with childbirth or a trained doula (childbirth support person) who is qualified in creating a safe space for you and your family.

Something you might not have control over is the nurse or nurses who are providing your care. One way that you can tip the scales in your favor is to be extra nice to the nurses from the moment you walk in.

Many times as a doula, when I'm home with women before going to the hospital, we spend time baking cookies or other treats so we can show up at the hospital and give these to the nurses to start off the relationship in a positive way. A box of chocolates or basket of fruit would also be very welcome and show the nurses that you want to get along with them and have respect for their hard work. Getting nurses on your side is pivotal in creating a supportive birth environment. Make sure that if you hire a

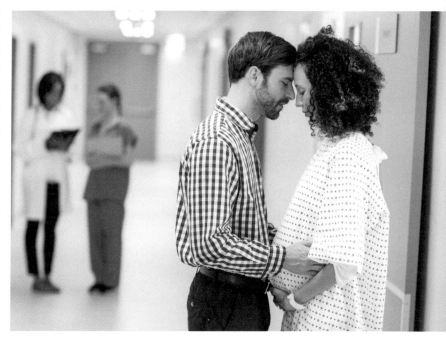

doula, that your doula has a primary objective of getting along with and being helpful to the nurses and doctors. Any contentiousness will undermine your goal of a peaceful and positive relationship with the nursing staff.

Optimizing Your Internal Environment

Create a way to feel safe in your body no matter what's going on outside. Trust the process of birth and your body's ability to give birth.

Practice a form of meditation or relaxation techniques that will help you stay present and in the moment. Remember that no matter what happens outside of you, you are in control of your mind, and your thoughts are related to how your body works. Having been a hypnotherapist for more than 21 years, I am a huge believer in using and practicing relaxation techniques and reprogramming our bodies to focus on the positive sensations that we feel. I do not believe that the ultimate goal of hypnosis is to have a pain-free labor; rather, it is to be able to observe the sensations we are feeling without the negative emotions that "pain" triggers. We will explore this topic in much greater detail in Chapter 10, Sensation Control.

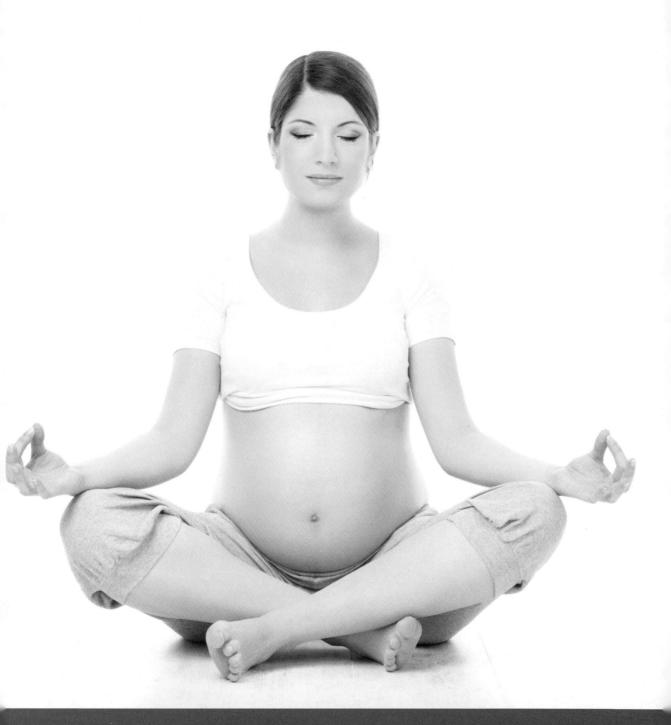

Chapter 7

LABOR AT HOME LONGER

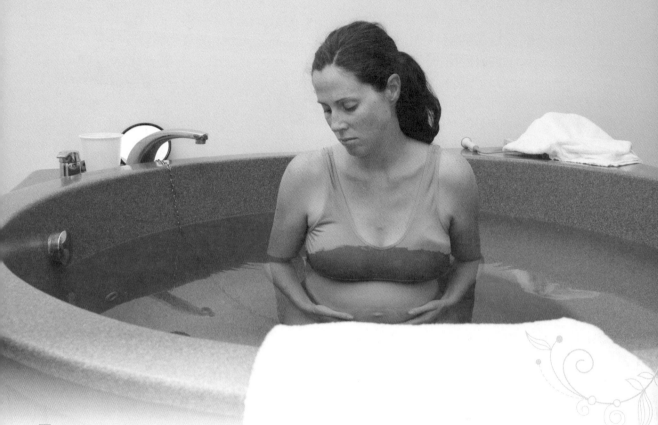

THE ONE CONSTANT ABOUT LABOR AND CHILDBIRTH IS THAT IT IS UNPREDICTABLE.

You may have heard things like, "The average first-time labor is 24 hours." There is really no way to tell how long your labor is going to be. Even if everyone in your family has had 12-hour labors, yours could be very different. Even though we can't predict how long labor will be, there are some universal signs that provide an indication of progression. Knowing these signs is important because many times women will go to the hospital very early in labor and get sent home because their labor is not very far along. This can be discouraging and upsetting for women and their families.

Also, if a woman is admitted to the hospital too early in her labor, she has a higher risk for unnecessary interventions, because typically women are less comfortable at the hospital and under pressure to show progression so as not to occupy a room that could be needed for another pregnant woman who is laboring more rapidly. Being at the hospital during the early parts of labor can lead to more interventions, less comfort during labor, and sometimes limited mobility that can impact fetal positioning and promote more contraction pain, leading to earlier use of pain medication and increased risk of cesarean.

Early labor is typically considered the time from when the cervix has not dilated at all until it has opened 3 to 4 centimeters. More progressive hospitals consider early labor as 0-6 centimeters. Early labor is the longest phase of labor for most women and is the most unpredictable in length. During this time, contractions are irregular but getting increasingly stronger and longer. They do not go away after resting or doing relaxing things like showering. They range from about 5 to 30 minutes apart and typically last around 30 to 45 seconds each. During this time, women experience a variety of sensations such as abdominal cramping or back pain. Many times these contractions start as menstrual-like cramps and build in intensity.

Active labor, traditionally, has been thought of as the time the cervix is dilating from four to eight centimeters. This is the time that hospitals prefer to admit laboring women. They like to see progression of about one centimeter per hour from this point on. If progression takes longer, interventions are often used. Active labor occurs when contractions are regular and more intense. They require a woman's concentration and range from three to five minutes apart, lasting approximately 45 to 75 seconds. At this point, the cervix is soft and very thin. Near the end of active labor, many women will feel pelvic and rectal pressure as they move into the next phase. The earlier method of assessing dilation assumes active labor begins at four centimeters. However, this assessment of dilation is beginning to change in many places.

As dilation progresses the baby moves down through the pelvis. When the baby gets to the middle of the pelvis, usually when the cervix is around 6 centimeters dilated, the baby encounters two small bones called the ischial spines protruding from the sides of the pelvis. This is one of the hardest places for the baby to navigate and sometimes can lead to a stall in labor progression. Because of this, many birth professionals now consider early labor to be from **0 to 6** centimeters dilation, meaning that the expectation to dilate one centimeter per hour doesn't begin until after 6 centimeters dilation, when the baby is through the ischial spines.

This is important, because if a woman is at four or five centimeters and is not dilating one centimeter per hour, hospitals may feel the necessity to augment her labor in order to speed it up.

Thinking about active labor as starting after 6 centimeters dilation would reduce the amount of intervention done by hospitals and decrease the cesarean rate.

Transition, is the next phase of labor, when the cervix is dilating from approximately 8 to 10 centimeters. This is typically the shortest and most intense part of labor. Contractions range from about 2 to 3 minutes apart and typically last 90 to 120 seconds. At this time, many women feel rectal pressure, like they have to have a bowel movement or urinate, especially at the peak of the contractions. It is also common for women to experience some nausea or shaking and possibly become either extremely focused or move into fight-or-flight response. The feeling of rectal pressure ultimately leads to an intense urge to push, resulting in the start of the **pushing phase** and **birth of the baby**.

It is important to talk to your care provider to see when they want you to come to the hospital. Many doctors and hospital midwives advise that you come to the hospital when the contractions are what we call 4-1-1. This means that the contractions are 4 minutes apart; they are at least 1 minute long AND they have been that way for at least 1 hour. Many times, observing contractions in this way helps women avoid arriving at the hospital too early. Knowing this, *it is important to be prepared to labor at home for potentially many hours*, so you don't get sent back home or admitted too early.

Note: Some hospitals are now using 3-1-2 instead of 4-1-1, meaning that the woman would wait to go to the hospital until contractions are 3 minutes apart, they are at least one minute long, and they have been that way for 2 hours.

HERE ARE SOME WAYS TO HELP YOU FEEL MORE COMFORTABLE STAYING AT HOME LONGER

Timing contractions

First of all, learn the correct way to time your contractions. As seen in the chart below, we time a contraction from the beginning of one contraction to the beginning of the next contraction. This is how far apart contractions are. The duration is from the beginning of the contraction to the end of the same contraction. There are many apps that will do this for you on a smart phone or a computer. This will save you time and energy. Don't feel like you need to log every single contraction. Just notice when the contractions seem to be getting more intense and closer together, and time them at that point.

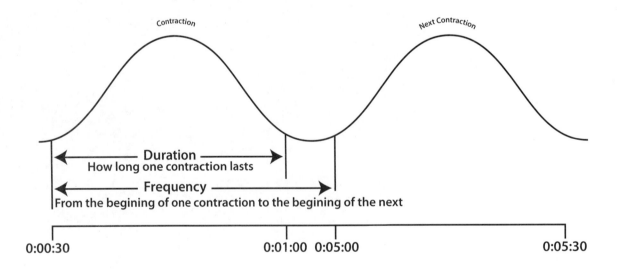

How to time a Contraction

Contraction   Next Contraction

Duration
How long one contraction lasts

Frequency
From the begining of one contraction to the begining of the next

0:00:30   0:01:00 0:05:00   0:05:30

Make a plan

If you spend your time in early labor focused on every contraction and nothing else, you'll end up going to the hospital much sooner than if you keep yourself occupied while remaining aware of your labor's progression. When I help women prepare for their labors, I will often ask them to create an early labor plan with suggestions of things that they may enjoy doing to help them stay occupied and engaged during early labor. Some possible early labor activities are baking, playing games, doing some yoga that feels good, meditation, taking walks, taking a bath or shower, cuddling or being intimate with your partner, slow dancing, watching a movie, listening to music, receiving a gentle massage and diffusing essential oils.

Comfort measures

It is important to be able to stay as comfortable as possible during this time to avoid experiencing more intensity than you need to, which could lead you to go to the hospital sooner.

SOME WAYS THAT YOU CAN ENJOY THIS TIME OF LABOR MORE ARE:

Sitting on a birth ball

Birth balls are very comfortable to sit on, because they mold to the pelvic area and allow pelvic movement during and between contractions. They are also nice to lean over, so you can relax in a way that is more conducive to optimal fetal positioning.

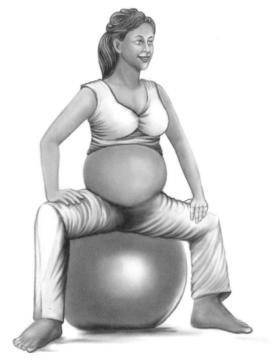

Hot sock or hot water bottle

Hot socks or hot water bottles are very comfortable for laboring women. The heat feels really good on contracting muscles and can reduce negative sensations by helping a woman focus on the pleasure of the warmth. A hot sock can easily be made at home by filling up a long sock with uncooked rice and tying off the end. These can be heated up in the microwave and stay warm for quite a while.

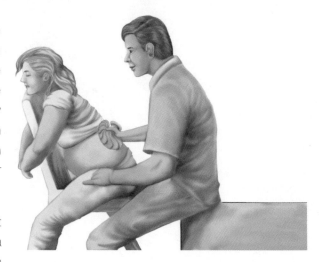

Note: be careful not to overheat the sock, or it will burn. Make sure that the sock is wrapped in a towel if it is too hot so as not to burn the woman using it.

Bath or Shower

Taking a bath or shower can decrease the sensation of labor contractions by up to 50 percent for many women. Occasionally, if too early in labor, a warm bath can slow things down, but it is a very effective tool once labor is established. Be aware that sometimes doctors do not want women to go into a bath after their water is broken, so please ask your health-care provider if this is the case.

Additional early labor ideas.

Other things to consider doing during early labor include massage, the rebozo and other optimal fetal positioning techniques. (See chapter 3)

REBOZO SIFTING

How to do it

Place a woven blanket or rebozo under woman's belly (like a hammock) while she is in a hands-and-knees position or on her knees resting over a birth ball. Partner stands above her and holds each side of the rebozo and gently lifts and shifts the rebozo back and forth a couple of inches. This should feel really good to the woman. Speed of the shifting can increase if comfortable. This technique can be done for a couple of minutes at a time in labor or in pregnancy.

Benefits:

- Relaxes the ligaments of the uterus, especially the broad ligament
- Relaxes mother
- Can speed up labor

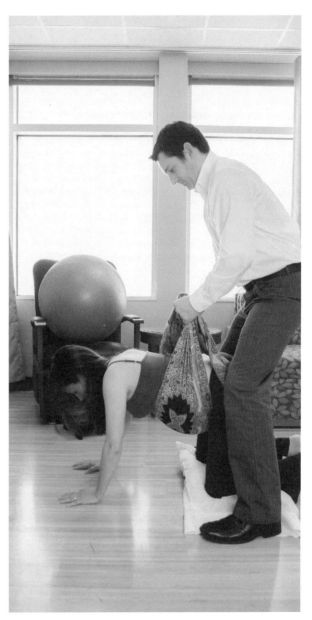

Spinning Babies

HERE ARE SOME TIMES IT MAY BE NECESSARY TO GO TO THE HOSPITAL EARLIER THAN WE HAVE DISCUSSED

If your doctor has asked you to come in for any reason

Some doctors or midwives like you to come in when your water breaks, or if you think your water might have broken, to assess your situation. At that point, they might send you home again or have you stay at the hospital. Other doctors will allow you to be at home with your water broken for many hours without needing to see you right away. Another reason a doctor might ask you to come in earlier is if you have another medical condition that needs to be assessed at the onset of labor.

Water breaking special circumstances

If your water breaks and it has any of the following characteristics, you will need to go to the hospital earlier:

- Green or brown tinged water
- Pieces of anything floating in the water
- Foul smell
- The water breaks with a big gush (call doctor right away)
- Known infection

Not feeling baby moving

If you are not feeling the baby move, call and let your doctor or midwife know. They will likely ask you to do a kick test by drinking some juice and lying on your left side and monitoring movement, or they may ask you to come in.

Bleeding

Sometimes, there may be light bleeding with labor. However, if the bleeding is heavy or has large clumps in it, call the doctor or midwife immediately and head to the hospital.

Mother's intuition

Always listen to your instincts. If you feel that something is not right, play it safe and go to the hospital, or call your doctor or midwife and let them know how you are feeling.

 kick test

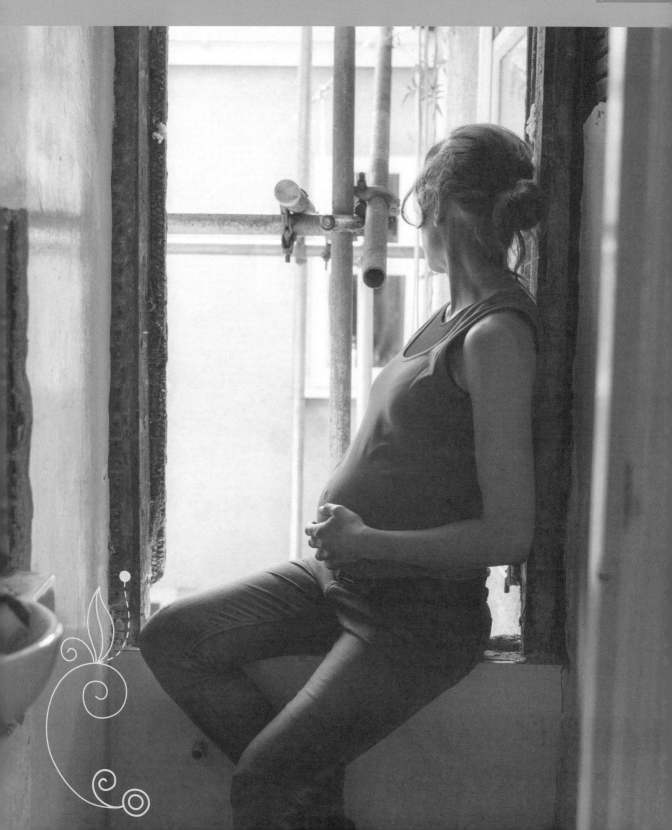

Chapter 8

AVOID EARLY EPIDURAL
AND OTHER INTERVENTIONS

THE EPIDURAL HAS BEEN REFERRED TO AS "THE CADILLAC OF ALL PAIN MEDICATION," BECAUSE IT IS SO EFFECTIVE IN REDUCING THE PAIN OF CHILDBIRTH.

Because of its reputation, some women will jokingly say they want to have an epidural even before they go into labor. Though in many cases epidurals are quite safe, it is a good idea to understand the risks and benefits of getting an epidural and how the timing of it may affect labor and childbirth.

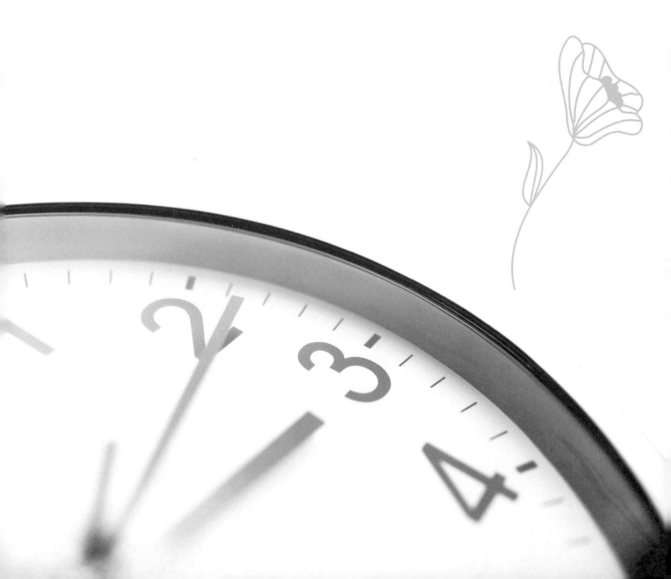

WHAT IS AN EPIDURAL?

There two types of pain medications that are commonly used during labor and delivery. The first is analgesics. The second is anesthetics, which includes epidurals.

Analgesics are narcotics that are commonly given as a shot into either a muscle or a vein. The most commonly used narcotic medications in labor and childbirth are Morphine,[15] Stadol, Fentanyl, Nubain and Demerol. These go directly into the mother's bloodstream and cross the placenta, affecting baby as well as mom. Because of this, analgesics are not given within a few hours of delivery of the baby, as they can affect the baby's respiration. The first thing the baby needs to do when he is born is to breathe! Analgesics given too close to time of delivery can cause the newborn baby to need breathing support or anti-narcotic drugs. Analgesics, in most cases, do not take the pain of labor away. However, they do take the edge off, enabling mom to rest more between contractions and relax tense muscles. The reason analgesics are sometimes used instead of epidurals is that they don't stay in the mom's system very long. The mom only feels the effects for about 45 minutes or so. This can be desirable because it means the mother will be able to have more mobility once the medication wears off, in contrast to having an epidural that will usually keep her in bed for the duration of her labor.

Epidurals are used to numb the body to take away the pain and some discomforts of labor contractions. An epidural is administered in the lower spine (usually in the vicinity of L4 and L5). After making sure the woman has been given intravenous fluids, the anesthesiologist will position the woman either sitting on the side of the bed with her back rounded, or less commonly in the United States, lying in the bed on her side. Her back will be washed with an antiseptic solution, and a sterile drape will be applied.

At this point, it is common for anesthesiologists to numb the area where the needle will be inserted, as the needle is long, thick and hollow. Once the area is numb, they will ask the woman to hold completely still with her back rounded and insert the needle into the epidural space surrounding the spinal column without puncturing the spinal column. They will then thread a small catheter through the needle and remove the needle keeping the catheter in place, and then tape the catheter to her back to prevent it from slipping. They will continue taping all the way up to her shoulder, where there will be a port to connect the catheter to continuous pain medication. The pain medication used in epidural anesthesia is a combination of narcotics and local anesthetics such as bupivacaine. Epidural anesthesia is generally very effective in reducing the pain of labor contractions, which is why the Centers for Disease Control report that more than 60 percent of women in the U.S. choose this option. Epidurals do not work the same way for every woman;

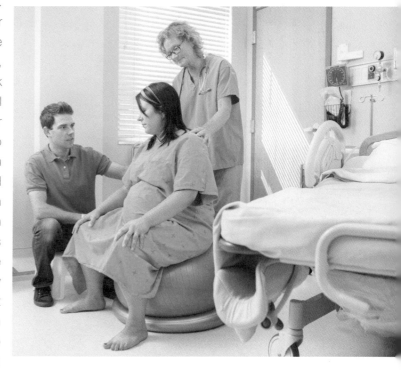

some women will have more sensation than others or have places where sensation remains. Most women will continue to feel pressure sensations though the majority of the "pain" is gone.

Epidurals work by blocking nerve impulses from the lower spinal segments. This reduces sensation and sometimes mobility in the lower half of a woman's body. Most of the time, women will still be able to move their legs but not walk around. Occasionally, the epidural will impact her mobility more extensively. Because of this reduced mobility, women are put in bed once the epidural has been administered, most commonly lying on their side. They need to switch sides regularly because the medication works with gravity; otherwise, over time, the lower side of her body gets more numb, and the upper side has more feeling.

For all of these reasons, once a woman has an epidural, she will be confined to the bed with an IV, a Foley catheter, a blood pressure cuff and fetal and maternal monitors. The IV provides access to administer any medications needed to augment her labor, as an epidural can slow down labor when given early in the process.[16] The Foley catheter is used to continually empty her bladder because she cannot get up to use the toilet and if the bladder gets too full, it can act like a balloon and hold the baby's head up in the pelvis. The blood pressure cuff is necessary because epidurals have been known to suddenly decrease blood pressure, making interventions necessary. The fetal and maternal monitors track the heartbeat of the baby with the mother's contractions to alert the medical staff to any fetal distress.

WHEN IS THE BEST TIME TO GET AN EPIDURAL?

One of the problems I have seen with women who go into their birth experience expecting to get an epidural is that they are not prepared for the amount of time that they have to labor without one. In the section above, we explored a few of the interventions that go along with getting an epidural. Because of these interventions and their propensity to interfere with the normal progression of labor, doctors don't like to give women epidurals before they are at least three centimeters dilated. This could take more than half of the time of her entire labor. When women are not prepared for this, they tend to feel the sensations of labor more powerfully and have a harder time coping with the intensity.

Some studies[17] indicate that if a woman gets an epidural before she is 4 centimeters dilated, the likelihood that she'll need a cesarean rises by 50 percent. Those same studies report that if she gets an epidural after 5 centimeters dilation, her chances of having a cesarean are the same as if she did not have an epidural. However, the epidural can still slow down progression. When labor progression is slowed due to the epidural, more interventions are needed to speed it back up, which can lead to other complications.

In my travels throughout the world, I have noticed that the amount of time women are allowed to labor varies greatly. Sometimes if a woman is in labor for too long, a cesarean is recommended. "Too long" in some circumstances could mean 48 hours, 24 hours, 12 hours, 6 hours or even less. So if a woman gets an epidural early and it lengthens her labor, she could be faced with getting a cesarean she may not have otherwise needed strictly because of time limits. My advice to women who want an epidural is to prepare to wait as long as possible before getting it by using comfort measures and relaxation techniques to allow the body to open up and give the baby the best chance to navigate the pelvis quickly and efficiently.

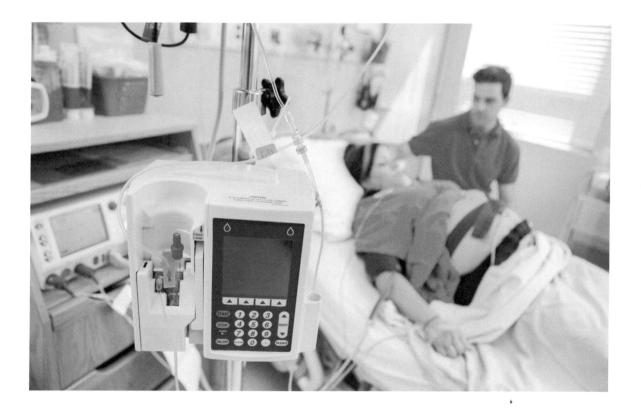

RELAXATION TECHNIQUES

PHYSICAL

Let's revisit the comfort measures from Chapter 7 in greater detail as they pertain to delaying an epidural.

Water

It is worth reiterating that using water can decrease the sensations of labor for some women by up to 50 percent. The pleasurable sensations of water actually reach the brain faster than pain sensations do. That's why when you're a kid and you fall down and scrape your knee and your mother kisses it, it actually makes it feel better, because the pleasure sensation of the kiss reaches the brain faster than the pain sensation of the scrape. This is also why heat and touch can be so effective in reducing the sensations of labor. Positive sensations like water and heat also bring on feel-good hormones such as endorphins or beta-endorphins, which act as powerful analgesics.

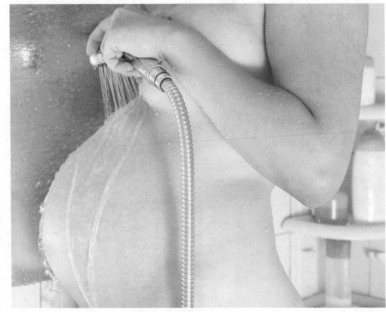

Movement

As we've discussed in the fetal positioning chapter, movement not only feels really good for a laboring woman, it also creates space and encourages the baby to get into a more favorable position for moving down through the pelvis. Our bodies are very intelligent and let us know the movements that are going to be most conducive for birthing by having those positions feel better than others. Change positions often; some movements that will likely feel good are forward leaning, sitting on a birth ball, walking, slow dancing with your partner, hip circles, and all-fours positions. If you are going to get an epidural, doing these positions first will give you a better opportunity for a less complicated vaginal delivery later.

Stay Upright

Along with the advice for movement, staying out of bed as much as possible in upright and forward-leaning positions is going to feel better for most women and help labor progression substantially. This is important because once a woman gets an epidural; she no longer has the option to be upright. I believe the main reason women get cesareans in greater numbers when they have epidurals early is that after they get an epidural, their movement is drastically limited, thereby creating a circumstance where babies don't have the space or opportunity to get into a good position for delivery. If a woman is in one position for a long time and her baby gets into a position that contributes to fetal distress, the baby does not have the opportunity to change that position as easily as if the mother were able to move around, creating space for the baby to resolve the malposition.

Birth Ball

The birth ball is a great way to stay in upright and forward-leaning positions while also enabling rest and relaxation. Revisit Chapter 7 for specific suggestions on how to use the birth ball.

Massage

For many women, massage during or between contractions can be enormously helpful. Make sure anybody touching you during labor is someone who will be sending you love and support through their touch. If somebody is feeling anxious or nervous, touch might be more of an irritation, even if the intention is good. Massage works best in labor on the lower back and hips as well as the neck and shoulders. If massage is not working for you, try heat from a hot sock or hot water bottle, as we talked about in Chapter 7.

Intimacy

Try turning down the lights and slow dancing with your partner or sitting between their legs on the bed, lying back against them. Just like water, being intimate increases positive sensations and endorphins, creating a feeling of safety and support as well as increasing oxytocin levels to keep labor going. Some of the most beautiful births I've attended are those in which the couple is in physical contact, holding each other and creating an intimate space during labor.

RELAXATION TECHNIQUES

EMOTIONAL

There are many things that will affect a woman's ability to maintain her stamina and emotional stability while waiting to get an epidural.

Music

Have you ever noticed how dramatically your mood can change when your favorite song comes on the radio? Music has the ability to help us to change our emotional state and is an amazing tool for laboring women. I encourage women to make a play list and bring it with them along with headphones or a speaker to help to change the atmosphere of the birthing room. Especially effective is playing inspiring music that encourages them to want to move or relax and also helps them feel safe.

Laughter

You may think that labor is the least likely time that you would find a woman laughing, but laughter actually helps release hormones that reduce negative sensations and increase positive ones. On many occasions, I have played board games with women in labor or watched a funny movie and have seen the power of laughter and its positive effects on her emotions.

Creating a safe environment

See Chapter 6 for a detailed explanation of ways that you can feel safe at a hospital.

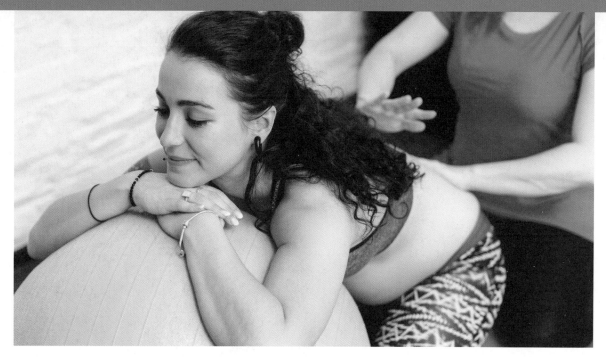

Doula support

As we discussed in Chapter 1, some statistics indicate that hiring a doula can reduce your chance of having a cesarean by 50 percent. Many people think that if they are planning on having an epidural, that they don't need a doula. But as we've discussed, much of labor is done before the epidural is given, and having a doula can be very helpful in allowing women to feel more comfortable so they can wait longer before getting the epidural.

Doulas can:

- provide emotional support
- suggest position changes
- keep the family informed about expectations and labor progress
- help with relaxation techniques to keep the mom's stress low
- assist with pushing
- provide immediate postpartum comfort and initial breast-feeding support

Meditation and sensation control

This is such an important aspect of avoiding an early epidural and reducing your chance of having a cesarean that it deserves it own chapter. See Chapter 10, Sensation Control, where we dive deeply into this topic.

Chapter 9

PELVIC OPENING

MOVEMENTS
SPECIFIC TO LABOR

The Bed icon indicates the positions can be done in bed!

REBOZO SIFTING

In labor, Rebozo Sifting can be done any time. However, it is especially useful to relax a woman when used between contractions during early labor. Use Rebozo Sifting if there is a lull in labor, especially around 5 to 7 centimeters.

YOGA

Yoga can be used in labor if it feels good. However, avoid inversions (any positions where the hips are above the heart) unless specifically using techniques that may help with malposition issues. Below are some times that different yoga positions can be helpful and comfortable.

Cat/Cow - *Any time during labor*

Doing Cat/Cow with contractions is even more helpful than doing it throughout pregnancy. Using gravity and movement, this position encourages a head-down baby to rotate in a way that allows the head to fit into the pelvis more easily.

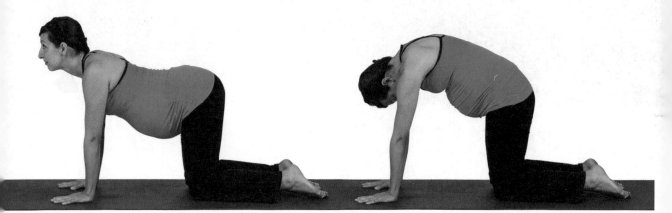
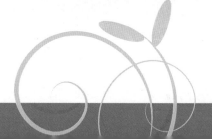

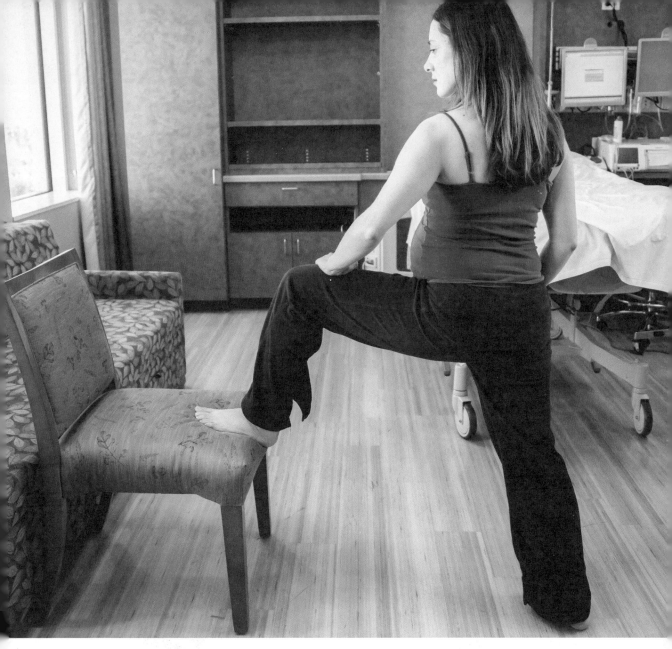

THERE ARE A FEW TECHNIQUES THAT CAN HELP YOU STAY PHYSICALLY BALANCED AND IMPROVE YOUR COMFORT DURING PREGNANCY AND BIRTH.

They are not all appropriate for all women, so check with your doctors before performing these exercises. *Carefully follow the guidelines that accompany each exercise.* Some of these can easily be done in bed, while others require a woman to have more mobility options. If you're at a facility where you're told you cannot get out of bed, pay special attention to the positions below with stars next to them.

Bound Angle - *Early labor*

This position is wonderful to do if your baby is high in the pelvis and having trouble moving down, as it opens up the pelvis' superior opening.

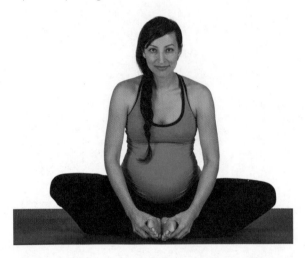

Child's Pose - *Any time during labor*

Child's Pose with knees wide and a couple of pillows under the torso can be a very comfortable position to rest in during early labor. It stretches the pelvic floor to help with any muscle tightness. If a woman has the center of her forehead resting on a pillow or her hand, she is activating a pressure point that encourages relaxation. Also, in this position the weight of the baby is away from the spine, giving the baby more space to move into a more conducive position for descending into or through the pelvis. Child's pose can be done during or between contractions. (See chapter 3 for more information on optimal fetal positioning).

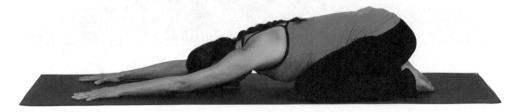

Seated Rocking - *Any time during labor*

This technique is one of my favorites for early and active labor. You may want to slightly elevate the hips on a blanket or thin pillow. This can also be done sitting on a birth ball next to the bed or in a rocking chair, though it is harder to set your own rhythm in a rocking chair. I also find it much easier to drop into a meditative state during rocking when I use music, so I recommend doing that. The rocking can be done with contractions, or just in between them, whatever is most comfortable for you. This works very well, especially if practiced 15 minutes a day during pregnancy, starting any trimester, the earlier the better!

See page 121 for detailed instructions

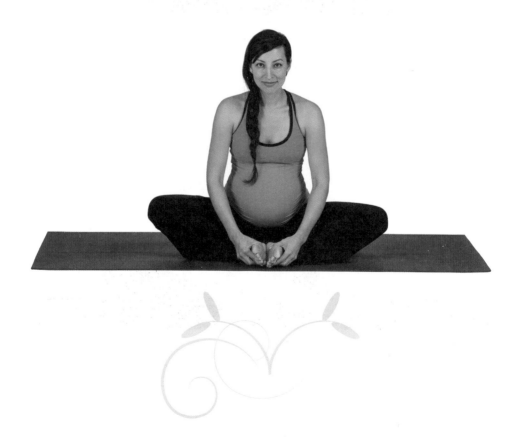

Seated Side Stretches - *Early labor*

These are great for releasing tension and helping a woman stay more relaxed in early labor. They're best done between contractions.

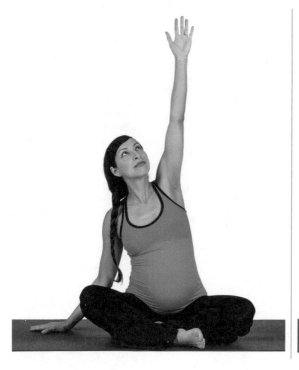
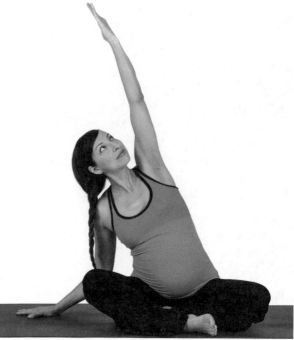

Anything that feels good!

Go ahead and practice some yoga in early labor, as long as it feels good. You may want to avoid inversion at this point except for a short downward dog if your body is asking for it.

Side Lying Release

Side Lying Release should be done in early labor if contractions are irregular and the baby is in the pelvis. This is a great technique to use if a labor stalls at 5 to 7 centimeters or later, as it can help release tension or torque in the pelvic floor, which can realign a baby who has a tipped head (asynclitic). See page 47

Psoas Release

Psoas Release can be done in labor if a baby is having trouble getting low or dropping into the pelvis. It helps the baby's head to move under the pelvic brim. The Walcher's technique also helps move the baby under the brim; have the woman lie down with a roll under the top of her thigh, where the thigh meets the buttocks, and let her legs dangle off the bed.

Inversions

Inversions can be helpful in labor if your labor pattern is not regular or symmetrical, if you are having slow progress, or hip or back pain that seems stronger than the uterus contraction pain. But do this only if you have permission from your care provider. Inversions help get the baby out of the pelvis so that he or she can have space to adjust positions. Inversions can be held through one to three contractions and repeated if needed.

Starting on hands and knees, place a pillow under the knees and come down onto your elbows so your seat is high in the air.

The Walcher's technique

PELVIC TILTS

Use pelvic tilts with contractions to help the baby rotate to an anterior position, or do them anytime that it feels good in labor. You can do these on all fours (Cat/Cow) or standing. Standing pelvic tilt can also be done with an abdominal lift (lifting the abdomen from the bottom during a contraction, releasing when the contraction ends) for about 10 contractions. Use this if there is prodromal labor to encourage labor to move along or if you are having back labor. Although pelvic tilts can be done any time, don't do the abdominal lift with normal labor or if you have a history of fast labors.

LUNGES

Lunges open the mid-pelvis where the ischial spines are. This is a part of the pelvis that can be hard for babies to maneuver, so opening up one side at a time can sometimes be very helpful. It is best to do the lunge when a baby is at zero station or lower, usually between 6 and 7 centimeters dilated (this is when the baby's head is already engaged in the pelvis). Lunges in labor work well when done with contractions, because this will help the baby turn and fit through the pelvis more easily. Do them if there is a stall in active labor to help the baby turn and fit through the middle pelvis.

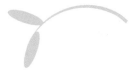

abdominal lift   prodromal labor, zero station

⬛ ROLL OVER (PENNY SIMPKIN TECHNIQUE)

Use the Roll–Over to get the most movement possible while in bed. Most positions can be used when a woman has had an epidural, but she will need help to do this! The Roll-Over is used mostly when a woman is at the end of labor and still not completely dilated, to help her dilation become complete.

Roll-Over (3 contractions in each position)

1. Hands and knees

2. Left side (you can start with either side), pillow between ankles and knees

3. Lying with belly pointing towards the bed. Left arm behind her, left leg straight (as much of a belly lying position as possible)

4. Open knee Child's Pose with hips elevated

5. Right side: Lying with belly pointing towards the bed. Right arm behind you, right leg straight (as much of a belly lying position as possible)

6. Right side pillow between ankles and knees

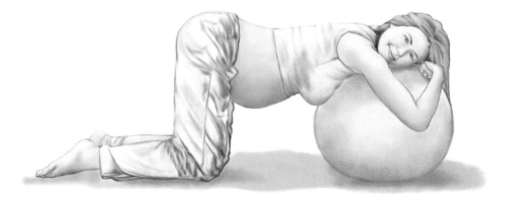

⬛ BIRTH BALL

There are many uses for birth balls in labor. They can be great for women who enjoy the hands-and-knees position but whose arms are tired. You can drape the upper body over the ball while maintaining the hands and knees position. Also, the ball can be next to a bed, and the woman can sit on it and rock her hips back and forth or in circles and lean forward on the bed. Balls also can be taken in the shower or tub and used to sit or lie on.

▣ SQUATS

Make sure both feet are flat on the floor and the belly is comfortable between the thighs. Sit on a bolster or block if more comfortable. Squatting while pushing and delivering the baby is one of the best positions to use, because it can speed up the descent of the baby reducing pushing time, relieve back pain, and it opens the inferior pelvic opening by up to 30 percent compared to lying on your back. This is also the position in which many women in the world give birth. Squats are great for the end of the pushing phase of labor. This pose is not advised if a woman is in labor and the baby is high in the pelvis. If the baby is low enough, this position helps the baby move down the birth canal because of the pressure the legs put on the belly. Squats can be quite intense if done during a contraction if the baby is too high, so if they don't feel good, don't do them. Squats can be modified to be more comfortable earlier in labor by doing the "dangle" where the partner sits in a chair and holds the woman up by the arms and she dangles in an elevated squat. Also a squat bar can be used near the end of pushing. Tie a sheet around it and have the woman pull on the sheet, or have her hang onto the bar with her hands or under her arms. Another squat position is having the woman face the partner, sitting on his lap with her bottom dangling down through his legs.

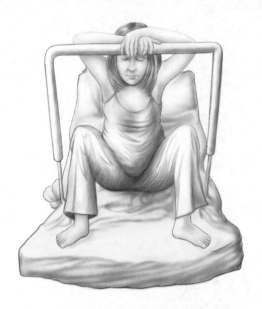

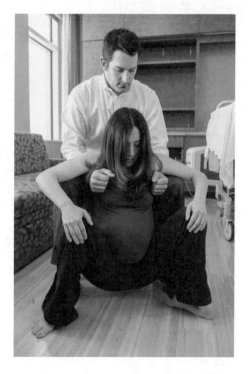

Chapter 10

SENSATION
CONTROL

BELIEVE IN YOUR BODY

I saved the most important chapter for last! In this chapter we will explore sensation. Everywhere I travel in the world, I ask women, "What is the first thing you think of when I say the word childbirth?" The vast majority of responses include one word: pain.

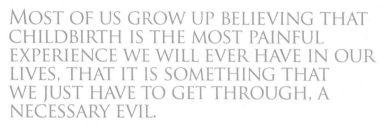

MOST OF US GROW UP BELIEVING THAT CHILDBIRTH IS THE MOST PAINFUL EXPERIENCE WE WILL EVER HAVE IN OUR LIVES, THAT IT IS SOMETHING THAT WE JUST HAVE TO GET THROUGH, A NECESSARY EVIL.

This impression is reinforced as we move into adulthood by the media depicting women screaming in labor. Stories we hear from other women who have given birth solidify this belief. Beliefs are powerful forces that can become self-fulfilling prophecies.

But what exactly is pain? This question is being researched in many prestigious pain centers right now. Think about if you had to describe what pain feels like to someone who has never experienced a sensation before. What would you say?

You might say, "It's a stabbing feeling or a burning feeling," but is all pain characterized that way? One thing that most people would agree upon is that pain is something to avoid; we spend most of our lives trying to evade it.

The reason for this is that pain is not merely a sensation; it is the only sensation that is both a "sensory and an emotional experience."[18] Pain is not only a physical sensation, like stabbing, burning, aching or pressure; it's a physical sensation that's accompanied by a negative emotional interpretation.

Most people think that labor is going to be very painful. This expectation makes it so that when a laboring woman begins to feel sensation during labor; she puts the name "pain" on that sensation which is immediately accompanied by a whole range of negative emotions. There are many sensations in labor that are quite positive, but most people don't experience them because they get trapped in the fear and expectation of pain.

Pain is very scary for most people. Our bodies respond to fear by reflexively tensing up to prepare for the pain sensation, which makes the sensation of pain more intense. As we get more afraid, our bodies tense up more. The fear-tension-pain cycle is the main reason that women scream during childbirth. Pain is driven and made considerably worse by the emotion of fear, whether it is fear of what is going on in their bodies, the awareness that they have to birth a baby and/or fear of the pain itself. The expectation of pain creates even more pain.

I had a doula client once who I helped prepare for her labor. I had her practice sensation control and some other techniques that you'll learn in this chapter. When it came time for her to have her baby, her doctor told her she needed to be induced. Unbeknownst to me, all of her co-workers had told her that if you are induced, you need an epidural because the pain is so much more intense. She went into the hospital to be induced, expecting the induction to cause even more pain than she would have had going into labor on her own. When they started her induction, I was not with her yet. She was only one centimeter dilated when she called me, frantically telling me I had to get over there because, in her words, "It hurts, it hurts so badly!" I rushed over to the hospital and found her sitting at the edge of her bed gripping the bed sheets with her hand as she moaned and cried. I knew by watching her, and by the fact that she was only one centimeter dilated, that the fear she was having played a big part in the amount of pain she was experiencing. So I sat down in front of her, placed my hands on her knees and looked her in the eyes. When she finished the next contraction, I said to her lovingly, "I can help you. Would you like my help?" And she said, "Yes." I said, "OK, here's what you need to do. For the next two contractions, I need you to become an observer of your body. Take yourself

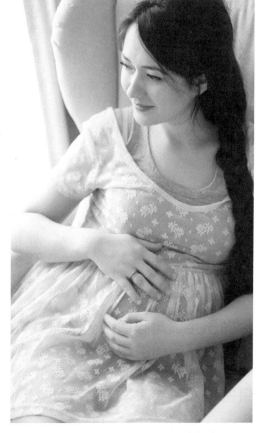

emotionally out of this experience for just two contractions. I want you to think about what it is you are actually feeling, but you are not allowed to use the word 'pain' to describe your sensation. You may notice some pressure or a squeezing. Identify the sensations without thinking or using the word 'pain.' You only have to do this for two contractions. Do you think you can?" She agreed she could do this. As the next contraction began, I saw her rocking gently back and forth with her eyes closed. When the contraction was over, she opened her eyes wide and looked at me and said, "It's just pressure!" This realization was very important to her because, without emotion behind it, the contraction was much more tolerable. As her labor progressed, the sensations never changed from pressure back to pain. The "pressure" got really intense, but it never felt painful, even at ten centimeters dilation. It was fear and not the contractions themselves that had made her contractions feel unbearable.

This might sound like I am saying that pain is all in your mind and that you can change it by simply changing your thoughts. And while it's true that changing your thoughts will change the sensations, it is far from simple for most people. The fear-tension-pain cycle creates a physiological response in the body. This response is what helps us stay alive when we are faced with danger. When we feel fear, our body releases hormones that speed up our heart rate, release adrenaline and bring all our energy to places in our body that are necessary for survival, so that we can run away or fight in response to the danger we are facing.

If we remove the fear from the sensations we are feeling, we can impact the hormonal response so that instead of releasing stress hormones, the body can release hormones that work to reduce pain and increase pleasure. These hormones are endorphins and beta-endorphins and can be stronger than morphine. If a woman is focusing on the things that feel good in her labor, such as the feeling of a contraction coming down or the feeling in between contractions when she is relaxed and comfortable, or the feeling of a warm compress or massage, being in water or being intimate with her partner, she can promote these feel-good hormones and drastically reduce her pain.

For most people, this process is not as easy as flipping a switch in their brain and telling them not to be afraid and to focus on the things that feel good rather than on the pain. Being able to do this takes

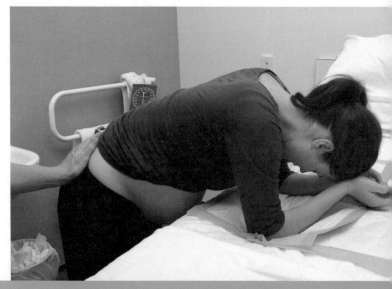

practice and work. We are so used to focusing on things that don't feel good and things we're afraid of, that we miss the positive sensations that accompany experiences like labor. Also, the protocols at most hospitals promote the concept that labor is painful. The nurses are instructed to come into the room and assess your pain levels every so often. They ask you to look at a series of pictures of smiley faces that start off happy and slowly move to crying. They inform you that the crying face is where you are headed and in so doing, reinforce your expectation that the sensations you are feeling are going to get unbearable.

In order to be able to change our thoughts during labor and focus on the positive sensations, it helps to practice doing this in daily life to create a habit of it, so that focusing on positive sensations and thoughts becomes automatic. When we have thoughts on a regular basis, those thoughts become more accessible to us and become our default way of thinking. This is physiologically happening in your brain! When we have a thought, it jumps from one synapse to another. The thoughts we have regularly bring those synapses closer together and thus make those thoughts more accessible. If we are constantly complaining and thinking about the things that don't feel good, negative thoughts will be dominant. We will then have to work very hard to have positive thoughts and focus on the things that feel good, because the positive-thought synapses are much further away from each other than the negative ones and therefore are less accessible.

Many of us think of ourselves as positive thinkers, convinced we are already in the habit of focusing on the positive. If you observe your thoughts and your language, you might notice a pattern of negative thinking that you had not known existed; this can impact you when it comes time to deliver your baby.

Here is where the practice comes in. There are several things that can drastically increase your chances of having a positive birth experience and help you increase the positive sensations of labor.

Practicing these things during pregnancy can help you with labor as well as with the postpartum period and your transition into motherhood.

The first part of this practice is observation of things that you say out loud. Notice if you catch yourself complaining a lot. There is a practice that Will Bowen talks about in his book, *A Complaint Free World*. He has people wear a bracelet, and every time they complain, they switch the bracelet to the other wrist. The goal is to keep the bracelet on one wrist for twenty-one days straight, because if you do something for twenty-one days, it becomes a habit. Pregnancy is a wonderful time for this practice, because you have a lot of motivation to change habits when you know it can help you immensely with labor and childbirth!

I'd heard about this challenge through a friend. I'd been teaching similar things for many years but had never seen the correlation between complaining and sensation control. This led to a pivotal moment one

day when I was travelling in China to conduct a yoga teacher training. It had taken me about 20 hours to get to the place where I was teaching. I had not slept and was very tired, and it was pouring rain. I arrived late at night at the retreat center where I was teaching and had to begin a nine-day training with 60 students the next morning. After a night of intense thunderstorms and only a few hours of sleep, I woke up and had to start teaching.

Before I left my room, I read a blog post from my friend who was doing the complaint-free challenge. I thought to myself, "I'm a yoga teacher. I don't complain very much, so I don't really need this challenge." But, as I walked out into the pouring rain, exhaustion took hold and I realized that all I wanted to do in that moment was to complain and that maybe this challenge did have some value for me! So instead of complaining, I opened my umbrella, turned to my husband and said, "It's going to feel so good when the sun comes out." In that moment, I felt sun on my face and imagined how it would feel. My whole day changed. I realized the power of our complaints. I started to think about all the things that felt good. I started to focus on my gratitude that I get to work with yoga teachers and pregnant women and help them create more positive birth experiences in the world. And yes, that day I changed my bracelet at least four times! But as I continued the practice, it got easier and easier. I stopped judging myself and started to notice the benefits of this challenge. Our thoughts and our words are powerful and can greatly impact the way we feel.

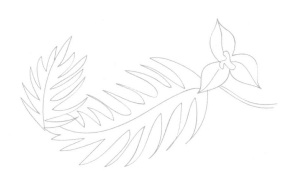

Wong-Baker FACES Pain Rating Scale, A Complaint Free World

HOW DO WE REDEFINE SENSATION?

In order to learn how to redefine sensation, one must learn to communicate with her body in a different way. They must first listen to their bodies and learn how to follow and interpret the signals they receive. Being aware of this need for connection is not enough to make it happen. It takes practice, and this practice takes different forms for different people. It is like learning another language, one with which you are vaguely familiar. You can pick out only a few words at first, but the more you immerse yourself in the language, the more fluent you become.

When women learn to connect to their own bodies, and the baby inside of them, they are able to redefine the sensations they are feeling and completely change their experience. A woman who is connected to her body understands that the energy she is feeling during childbirth is a powerful and dynamic force that she's creating from deep within herself so that she can birth her baby. She knows that no outside force is exerting pain upon her. Even when labor is augmented, it's her own body, her own self, creating an incredible amount of energy to give birth, to assist her baby into the world. Women have the ability to tap into this force and work with it instead of fighting it. When women are able to do this, they realize that they're not a victim of their birth experience and their bodies, but a participant in a miraculous experience!

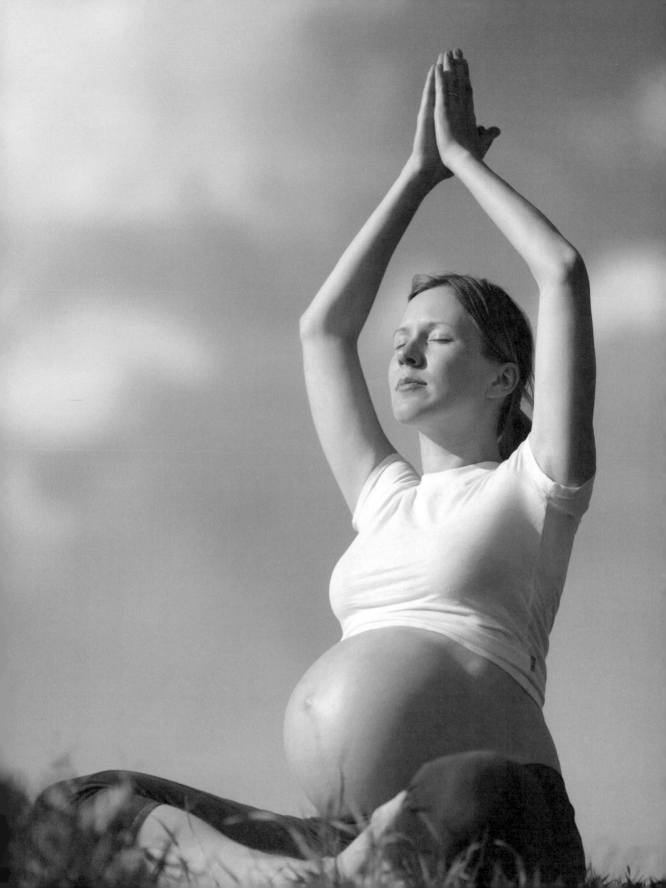

Here are some things you can practice to increase your connection with your body and help you become fluent in its language.

Prenatal Yoga

The sequence as described in Chapter 4 not only helps with fetal positioning, body discomforts, releasing endorphins, staying present in your body, and connecting with and moving with your baby, it's also a wonderful way to identify and focus on positive sensations. Yoga is a fantastic way to learn to communicate with your body on a deeper level, connecting your breath to your movements. Observing the way your body responds to different poses or positions can be so valuable. Making these practices part of your everyday life and bringing awareness into every sensation in your body is very helpful.

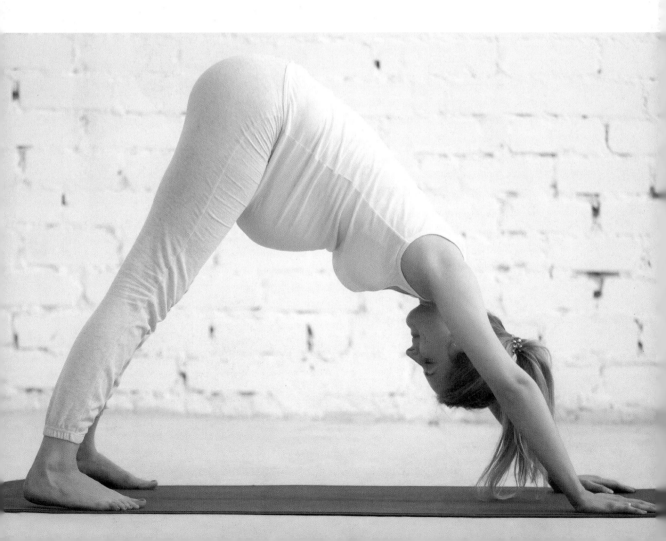

Rocking

This is one of the most effective ways to use relaxation in labor. This practice is very beneficial, as it not only creates a deep meditative state but also creates space for the baby to move into a more conducive position for labor and, ultimately, delivery. Your body feels much better, generally, when you're moving in labor. If practiced during pregnancy, rocking can bring on a deep trance state very quickly. By allowing the baby to find a good position to come down, rocking can speed up labor. Practice rocking three different ways to find the way that works best for you – first, sitting on a folded blanket cross-legged; second, on a birth ball; and third, standing. If you have access to a rocking chair, which many hospitals have, this would be another option.

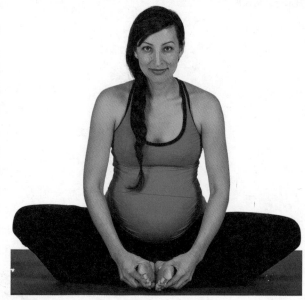

1. Make sure you are in a comfortable position.

2. Keep your spine long and as you inhale, rock your body forward, leading with your heart space, taking the entire inhalation.

3. As you exhale, rock back using the entire exhalation. At the end of the rock, you can round the back slightly, holding on to your knees with your hands.

4. Lengthen the spine as you begin your next inhalation.

5. Make sure you keep the rocking moving with your breath, all the way forward and all the way back.

6. It may seem counterintuitive, but rock all the way forward and all the way back. Don't allow the movements to get shorter or smaller as you relax. It is the repetition of this larger flowing movement connected to the breath that induces a deep meditative state. Practice this until your rocking feels automatic. You will soon feel that you don't have to try to rock; it just happens. Practice with music that will enhance your trancelike mood. Bring this music with you to the hospital or birth facility to help you effectively use rocking while in labor.

Take a walk

Using walking as a moving meditation, become an observer of your body and notice all of the sensations you feel, focusing on the positive ones. Start at your feet; notice your feet touching the ground, the rhythm of your steps, the feeling of air on your skin and in your hair; focus on your breath and how it propels you forward. Exhale and feel your body relax. Notice how your body feels after a block or two to have the muscles in your legs working; it can feel so good to use your muscles. After a few blocks, stop and lean against a tree or just stand or sit still and close your eyes; connect with your heart pumping blood to every part of your body. Connect to your breath moving oxygen, feeding your body and your baby. Take a sip of water and enjoy the thirst being quenched.

Take a piece of ice and hold it in your hand

Without using the word "pain," analyze the sensations you are experiencing; notice them as if they were new and interesting. Resist the temptation to put the ice down, and instead take a few deep breaths. Relax different parts of your body as you exhale and see how this changes the sensations you're feeling.

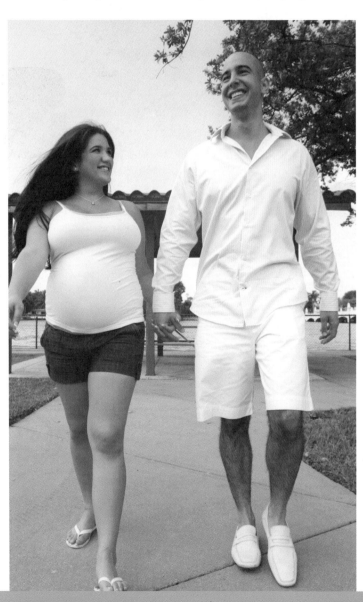

Lean against the wall with your feet away from the wall so that when you bend your knees, your knees are over your ankles.

Bring your arms up so they are parallel to the ground. Relax your shoulders and slide your back down the wall until your thighs are parallel to the ground. Hold this position for three breaths. During each breath, emphasize your exhalation by relaxing another part of your body that does not need to be tense. Now take three more breaths before coming out of the pose.

The Complaint Free Challenge

The Complaint Free Challenge described earlier, is one of the most powerful tools I've found to help change the neural pathways we create by negative thinking. This is an important first step along with prenatal yoga that can lead to more positive birth experiences. Beyond that, it can help prepare you for motherhood and the demanding challenges you face directly after having your baby. Pregnancy is the perfect time to start this practice because you have more motivation than at almost any other time in your life. As well as preparing you for labor and motherhood, you'll notice yourself focusing on the positive things about pregnancy, and you'll enjoy your pregnancy much more. The work you do in this challenge (and it will take some work and commitment) will have long-term effects including remembering pregnancy as a wonderful experience. This is an incredible way to begin the lifelong relationship you will have with your child.

Doing these exercises once or twice is a good start, but accessing the benefits of these techniques during labor takes practice (think about when you learned to ride a bike). I recommend doing the ones that feel good at least a few times a week. I also recommend practicing with an audio relaxation so that you get used to what it feels like to have your body relaxed. I've included a free audio download of sensation control for pregnancy and childbirth on the accompanying website.

There are so many more beneficial practices that have been used by women over the years to help birth feel more comfortable and even enjoyable! I've listed many of them with links on the accompanying website. My favorites are *Orgasmic Birth* by Debra Pascali-Bonaro and the research from the HeartMath Institute about the connection between one's breath and heart. Please check the links to their material!

audio download of sensation control, *Orgasmic Birth* by Debra Pascali-Bonaro, HeartMath Institute

FINAL THOUGHTS

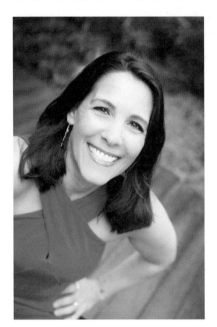

We all want birth to be a beautiful experience. We want our journey into motherhood to be one that teaches us how strong and capable we are. We want to feel as though the birth of this baby that we love so much is a positive experience, but the one constant in childbirth is that it is unpredictable. Sometimes, even if you use every tool available to you, you will still end up needing a cesarean. My goal in writing this book is not to say that cesareans are never appropriate, as I believe strongly that sometimes they are absolutely necessary. Instead, my intention is to empower you to play an active roll in your birth experience by encouraging you to get to know your body in a new way.

I BELIEVE ALL WOMEN SHOULD BE ENCOURAGED AND PREPARED TO GO INTO THE EXPERIENCE OF PREGNANCY AND BIRTH FEELING CONFIDENCE IN THEIR BODIES AND THEIR ABILITY TO BRING THEIR BABIES INTO THE WORLD WITH STRENGTH AND JOY, ALLOWING THE EXPERIENCE TO BE TRANSFORMATIVE AND BEAUTIFUL.

If a woman goes into childbirth physically and mentally ready, having practiced techniques and prepared her body for the experience, then even if the birth is long, or she ends up having a cesarean, in most cases, she will feel so much more at peace with the outcome.

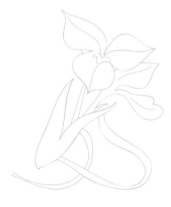

GLOSSARY OF TERMS

Bikini-cut Cesarean

A method of cesarean surgery using a horizontal incision just above the pubic area.

Cesarean

This describes the use of surgery to deliver a baby. Also referred to as a C-section or cesarean delivery. A cesarean is performed by the surgeon making an approximately 15cm incision (either horizontal, vertical, or both) through the mother's lower abdomen. The uterus is opened through a second incision, and the baby delivered. Incisions are then stitched closed. The surgery typically lasts between 45 minutes to an hour.

Doula

A non-medical birth companion, coach, and general support for a woman before, during, and after childbirth. Doulas can provide physical, emotional, and informational support to mothers as well as their families if needed.

Episiotomy

A surgical incision of the perineum, usually performed during the second stage of labor to enlarge the opening for the baby to pass through.

Gestational Diabetes

A condition in which a pregnant woman, without diabetes, develops high blood sugar levels.

Gut Microbiota

The complex community of microorganisms that live in the digestive tract of humans.

Hysterectomy

The surgical removal of the uterus. Depending on circumstances, the cervix, ovaries, fallopian tubes or other surrounding structures may also be removed.

Kick Test

A method to record fetal activity in the later stages of pregnancy.

Maternal Transfusion

This is the process of giving blood to the mother during childbirth.

Midwife

A birth professional, specializing in pregnancy, childbirth, women's sexual and reproductive health, and newborn care. Midwives can either be Certified Nurse Midwives and work in hospitals or birth centers or Homebirth Midwives.

Moxibustion

Traditional Chinese Medicine therapy consisting of burning dried mugwort (herb) near a particular point on the body.

Oxytocin

A hormone produced in the hypothalamus and released by the pituitary. Important in bonding, sexual reproduction, and during and after childbirth. Oxytocin is released during labor as well as with nipple stimulation during breastfeeding, contributing to mother-child bonding and continued milk production.

Pitocin

Synthesized oxytocin used to cause contraction of the uterus in order to start labor, speed up labor, or to stop bleeding after delivery.

Placental Abruption

A dangerous condition where the placenta detaches, either partially or completely, from the uterus, depriving the baby of oxygen, which can lead to the need for immediate delivery or bed rest.

Placenta Praevia

A condition in which the placenta is covering or partially covering the cervix. This is often diagnosed early in pregnancy but as the uterus grows the placenta moves with it upwards and away from the cervix. If the placenta is still partially covering the cervix in the third trimester the woman will not be able to deliver her baby vaginally and must have a cesarean.

Preeclampsia

A condition that is diagnosed when a woman has elevated blood pressure and protein in her urine. Symptoms can include, headaches, blurred vision, swelling of hands and feet, high blood pressure and protein in the urine.

Prodromal Labor

In a prodromal labor, the early phase of labor is prolonged with contractions that do not increase in intensity. Prodromal labor can tire a woman out and use up the energy she will need for active labor and delivery.

Prostaglandin

A group of compounds with hormone-like effects, pivotal in cervical ripening.

Shoulder Dystocia

When labor is obstructed after the delivery of the head, and the shoulders of the infant cannot pass below the pubic bone.

Thromboembolic Disease

When a blood clot forms in a vein and then dislodges to travel in the blood. Most commonly occurs in the deep veins of the legs or pelvis. Blood flow can be limited by the clot, causing pain and swelling in the leg.

TOLAC

Trial of labor after caesarian (TOLAC). An attempted vaginal birth in a patient who has previously had a cesarean. It may result in a vaginal birth or another cesarean.

Ultrasound

The medical use of sound waves to create real-time visual images of the developing embryo or fetus in the mother's uterus.

VBAC

Vaginal birth after Caesarean section (VBAC)

Water Breaks

When the amniotic sac ruptures and releases amniotic fluid. Normally occurring at full term, either at the beginning or during labor. Also referred to as the rupture of membranes (ROM). When done by a medical professional it is referred to as Artificial Rupture of Membranes (AROM).

Zero Station

When the baby's head is level with the ischial spines of the pelvis, also known to be "engaged". Fetal decent is measured from -5 to +5. Each number is about 1 cm of distance.

FOOTNOTES

1. http://apps.who.int/iris/bitstream/10665/161442/1/WHO_RHR_15.02_eng.pdf

2. https://www.ncbi.nlm.nih.gov/pubmed/18378742

3. http://www.acog.org/Patients/FAQs/Cesarean-Birth-C-Section#complications

4. https://www.ncbi.nlm.nih.gov/pmc/articles/PMC2475575

5. https://www.ncbi.nlm.nih.gov/pubmed/18352976

6. https://www.ncbi.nlm.nih.gov/pmc/articles/PMC3864895

7. http://www.cdc.gov/nchs/data/nvsr/nvsr64/nvsr64_04.pdf

8. http://www.acog.org/Patients/FAQs/Vaginal-Birth-After-Cesarean-Delivery-Deciding-on-a-Trial-of-Labor-After-Cesarean-Delivery

9. http://www.ncbi.nlm.nih.gov/pmc/articles/PMC3489119

10. http://www.lamazeinternational.org

11. http://www.ncbi.nlm.nih.gov/pmc/articles/PMC3226811 & http://journals.lww.com/greenjournal/Abstract/2013/06000/_Therapeutic__Bed_Rest_in_Pregnancy__Unethical_and.23.aspx

12. Depending on the country, situation and specific doctor protocols, the timing of induction can vary. In the US, it is recommended to allow women to wait until 42 weeks to deliver if there are no other complications; in some countries it is common to induce much earlier.

13. Possible negative side effects of ingesting castor oil include diarrhea, abdominal cramping, nausea and vomiting. Some medical professionals are also concerned that ingesting castor oil might increase the risk of the baby having its first bowel movement in utero.

14. www.ncbi.nlm.nih.gov/pubmed/21280989

15. Morphine will likely only be given to women when they are experiencing prolonged periods of contractions that are not resulting in dilation or labor progression (prodromal labor) because the effects last much longer than other narcotics (five hours in mom, eight hours in baby).

16. Epidurals have been known to slow down labor as well as speed it up, depending on the circumstances.

17. https://www.mdedge.com/obgyn/article/54868/obstetrics/early-epidural-doubles-c-section-risk-after-induction

18. http://www.iasp-pain.org/files/Content/ContentFolders/Publications2/ClassificationofChronicPain/Part_III-PainTerms.pdf

OTHER OFFERINGS BY JENNIFER MORE

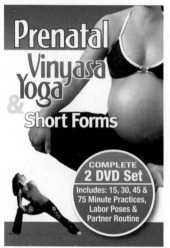

Prenatal Vinyasa Yoga offers a complete, safe, and active workout for all 3 trimesters and prepares you, your body and your baby for childbirth and postpartum recovery. This 2 DVD set provides you the most flexibility to tailor your yoga practice to meet your busy schedule and your energy level. It Features: 15, 30, 45 & 75 Minute Practices: Choose the length of your practice each day based on how much time you have and how your body is feeling. Each practice is different, so you won't get bored. 5 & 15 Minute Relaxations: Prepare your mind and body for labor by training your body to relax using this 5 minute relaxation, a great way to end your yoga practice. Safe Modifications for all 3 Trimesters: All 3 trimesters are modeled so you can modify your practice as your baby grows and your body changes. 10 Minute Partner Routine with Doug Swenson: Connect with your partner and baby using this informative and fun partner yoga segment. Bonus Labor Poses: Yoga can be really helpful in labor and childbirth, learn some tips for bringing yoga into the birthing process.

DVD   dolphinmethod.com/PrenatalVinyasaYogaDVD
Streaming/DL vimeo.com/ondemand/prenatalvinyasayoga &
                  vimeo.com/ondemand/prenatalvinyasayogasf

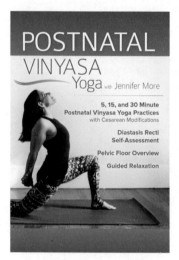

Postnatal Vinyasa Yoga has been carefully crafted to allow a new mom the opportunity to resume her yoga practice slowly, starting with the 5 minute, getting back on your mat practice. This practice is designed to get her back in touch with her body so she can safely resume her yoga practice while sending healing energy to the space where her baby lived for all those months. As a new mom it is difficult to find time to fit yoga in, this is why we have created a 15 and a 30 minute practice. Finding 15 minutes a day to do yoga is easy and she will notice the huge difference it will make. Just 15 minutes a day of making time for herself and the healing of her body, will contribute to more positive moods, more and energy during the day, becoming a stepping stone to reclaim her health and fitness. After making the 15 minute practice part of her routine, she will be able to integrate the 30 minute practice, this is where she will really start to see the benefits in her body, energy levels, strength and stamina. Eventually, with these two practices, she will feel ready to return to her regular yoga practice in a safer and more comfortable way.

DVD   dolphinmethod.com/PostnatalVinyasaYogaDVD
Streaming/DL vimeo.com/ondemand/postnatalyoga

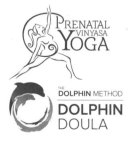

Prenatal Yoga, Yoga, and Doula Trainings with Jennifer More

Jennifer travels extensively, bringing Prenatal Vinyasa Yoga and Doula trainings to many locations around the World.

Schedule   dolphinmethod.com/trainings-workshops